THE CRUELLEST MILES

THE CRUELLEST MILES

The Heroic Story of

Dogs and Men

in a Race Against an Epidemic

Gay Salisbury & Laney Salisbury

BLOOMSBURY

First published in Great Britain 2003

Copyright © by Gay and Laney Salisbury 2003

The moral right of the author has been asserted

Bloomsbury Publishing Plc, 38 Soho Square,
London W1D 3HB

A CIP catalogue record for this available from the British Library

ISBN 0 7475 6061 7

10 9 8 7 6 5 4 3 2

Typeset by Hewer Text Ltd, Edinburgh
Printed by Clays Ltd, St Ives plc

All papers used by Bloomsbury Publishing are natural, recyclable
products made from wood grown in sustainable, well-managed forests.
The manufacturing processes conform to the environmental
regulations of the country of origin.

to Dorothea Boothe

Contents

Authors' Note   IX

Map of Alaska   XIV

Map of the Route of the 1925 Serum Run   XVI

PROLOGUE Icebound   3

1   Gold, Men, and Dogs   11

2   Outbreak   33

3   Quarantine   47

4   Gone to the Dogs   59

5   Flying Machines   79

6   Hunters of the North   111

7   The "Rule of the 40s"   137

8   Along the Yukon River   153

9   Red Tape   171

10   The Ice Factory   195

11   Cold Glory   213

12   Saved!   227

EPILOGUE: End of the Trail   243

Appendix A   257

Appendix B   263

Acknowledgements   265

Source Notes   269

Selected Bibliography   293

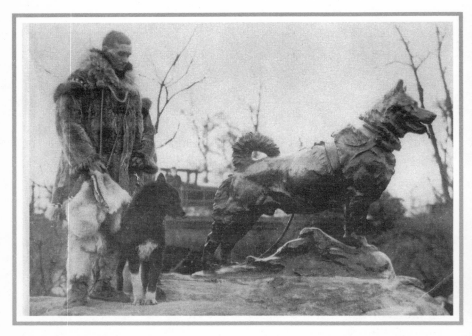

Gunnar Kaasen and lead dog Balto at the unveiling ceremony of Balto's statue in New York City's Central Park, December 16, 1925. The inscription at the base of the statue reads "Dedicated to the indomitable spirit of the sled dogs . . . ENDURANCE FIDELITY INTELLIGENCE."

(Photograph courtesy of Brown Brothers)

Authors' Note

Most of us find it impossible to resist the face of a friendly dog, or the details of a good dog story, and the story of dogs and men racing serum to save the children of Nome from diphtheria in 1925 was the greatest dog story ever told. Proof of this can still be found in Central Park in New York City where every year thousands flock to find the statue of a dog.

Balto was the dog who led the last relay team into Nome in 1925 under blizzard conditions, a feat that made him the world's most famous dog, next to the movie star Rin Tin Tin. Admiring dog lovers of New York who followed the extraordinary exploits of the dogs and men in the newspaper headlines commissioned a larger-than-life-size sculpture of Balto that was erected in December 1925, a short distance off Fifth Avenue near the entrance to the Children's Zoo. The plaque on the granite outcropping on which Balto stands dedicates the statue to the "indomitable spirit" of the sled dogs who ran to Nome: "ENDURANCE FIDELITY INTELLIGENCE."

We are first cousins, who both grew up in the New York area and were among the millions of children who loved to climb atop Balto whenever we played in Central Park. The great affection that children have for Balto is plainly visible. The bronze surface has been polished down to a gold sheen in places where children have petted his head, rubbed behind his ears, and climbed upon his back. The caretaker of the Central Park Conservancy estimates that the statue has lost a quarter inch in size during the many years that children have been riding on Balto's back. Though we knew no more about Balto than any other kids, we had heard frightful stories about diphtheria. One story in particular haunted us as children.

Our grandfather Dr. Edward Salisbury, a noted specialist in tropical diseases, was a physician at a rural outpost on the shore of the Caribbean Sea in eastern Costa Rica, where our fathers grew up together in the 1930s. When Gay's father, John Salisbury, was four years old, he contracted diphtheria, and our grandfather found himself with no antitoxin on hand, and none available anywhere in the entire country—the identical situation that Nome's only physician had faced less than nine years earlier. John's condition was so serious that everyone expected him to die within hours. The hospital nurse, Dorothea Boothe—to whom this book is dedicated—never left his side. At the last moment, however, Dr. Salisbury and his pilot flew to Panama, where they located a fresh supply of serum and, battling a severe tropical storm, arrived back at the remote hospital in time to save the child. No matter how many times we heard the story from our grandfather, grandmother, or from Dorothea herself (a woman for whom our family had the deepest love and respect), the most chilling details were that before the antitoxin arrived the priest had already administered the last rites, and the workers had constructed a child's coffin, less than four feet long, in preparation for the funeral.

The inspiration for this book came when we read an eloquent obituary in *The New York Times* of Edgar Nollner, the lone surviving 1925 musher, who died in January 1999 at the age of ninety-four. "Hero in Epidemic," read the headline, though the *Times* explained that Nollner always claimed that the twenty-four-mile stretch he mushed, in a blizzard so thick he could not even see his dogs, was "simply a day's work." According to the *Times*, Nollner was the last link to "one of the great cliffhangers of the 20th century, one that held a nation in white-knuckled thrall for more than a week in 1925 as the world wondered whether a supply of life-saving serum would make it to icebound Nome, Alaska, in time." Now the story was becoming a "fading memory," but Nollner had once helped to "carve a legend in the snow."

No roads have ever led to Nome, Alaska, a small community of about four thousand people on the coast of the Bering Sea, 2 degrees south of the Arctic Circle. For more than a hundred years, since its birth during the gold rush of the 1890s, Nome has been one of the most isolated communities on earth. Nome is icebound by a frozen ocean for at least seven months each year. "We are prisoners in a jail of ice and snow," one newspaper editor lamented in November 1900. In good weather, airplanes now link Nome to the rest of the outside world in any season, but still there are no roads that go anywhere, and even today driving to Nome is about as practical as driving to Hawaii. Unless, that is, you're standing behind a team of dogs.

Every March the nearly 1,200-mile Iditarod Trail Dog Sled Race takes place from Anchorage to Nome. Billed as "The Last Great Race on Earth," the Iditarod is a dash across the Alaska wilderness that combines elements of the Kentucky Derby and the Daytona 500. It features the world's fastest dogs and dog drivers in a grueling contest of skill, speed, and endurance. Organized in 1967 by Alaskans who wanted to preserve the traditions of dog mushing, the point of the Iditarod was to ensure that dog teams would always run along the trails of Alaska. A salute to Alaska's pioneers who connected isolated communities, the race was also intended to keep alive the memory of the most heroic dogsled race in history, the 1925 diphtheria serum run to Nome.

Numerous children's books have been written about Balto and the serum run—it was even the subject of a popular animated movie by Steven Spielberg—yet the only previous history of the events of 1925 was a fine book written nearly forty years ago, Kenneth A. Ungermann's brief account, *The Race to Nome.* In the years since, government documents, new oral histories, family records, medical archives, newspaper accounts, and unpublished photographs have surfaced, all of which have been instrumental in providing the complete story of what happened during those crucial six days in 1925 when the world was pulling for the dogs. The true story is more tragic and inspiring than any child could imagine, and it begins where the Iditarod ends, on the icebound shore of the Bering Sea.

"He who gives time to the study of the history of Alaska, learns that the dog, next to man, has been the most important factor in its past and present development."

—ALASKA JUDGE JAMES WICKERSHAM, 1903

"There was no line of retreat, no going back and covering the same ground twice."

—FRIDTJOF NANSEN on naming his expedition *Fram* to mean "Forward"

"Well, all I know about dogs is not much, but when I was up in Alaska . . . their whole existence tangles around dogs . . . the backbone of the arctic is a dog's backbone."

—WILL ROGERS's last column, recovered from the wreck of his fatal plane crash in Alaska, August 1935

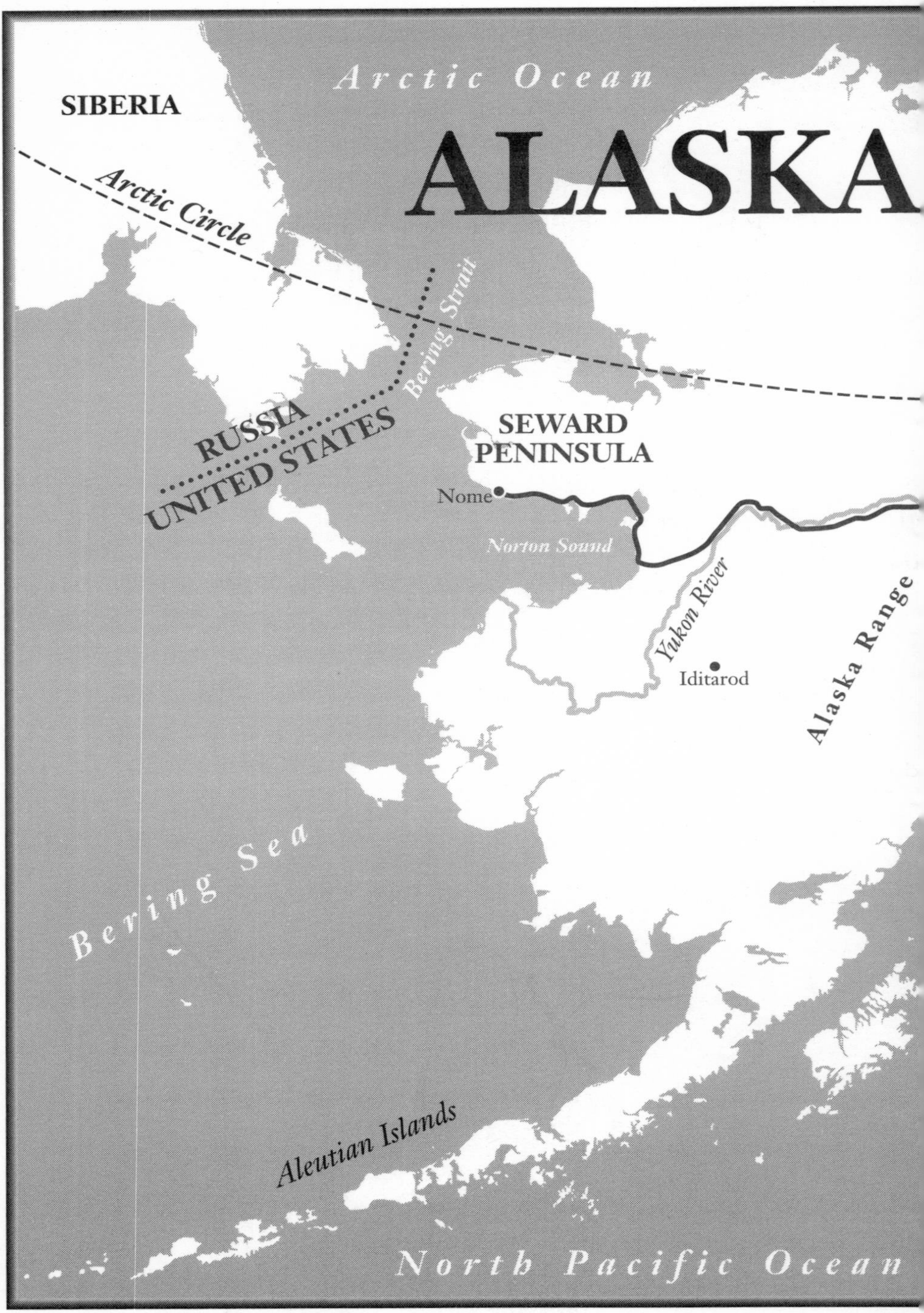

Arctic Ocean
SIBERIA
ALASKA
Arctic Circle
Bering Strait
RUSSIA
UNITED STATES
SEWARD
PENINSULA
Nome
Norton Sound
Yukon River
Iditarod
Alaska Range
Bering Sea
Aleutian Islands
North Pacific Ocean

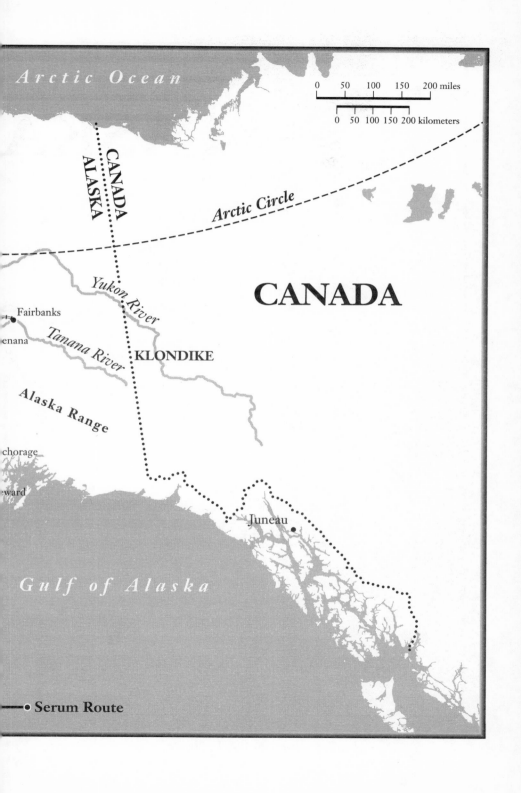

Arctic Ocean

0 50 100 150 200 miles

0 50 100 150 200 kilometers

Arctic Circle

CANADA
ALASKA

Yukon River

CANADA

Fairbanks

enana

Tanana River **KLONDIKE**

Alaska Range

:horage

:ward

Gulf of Alaska

Juneau

Serum Route

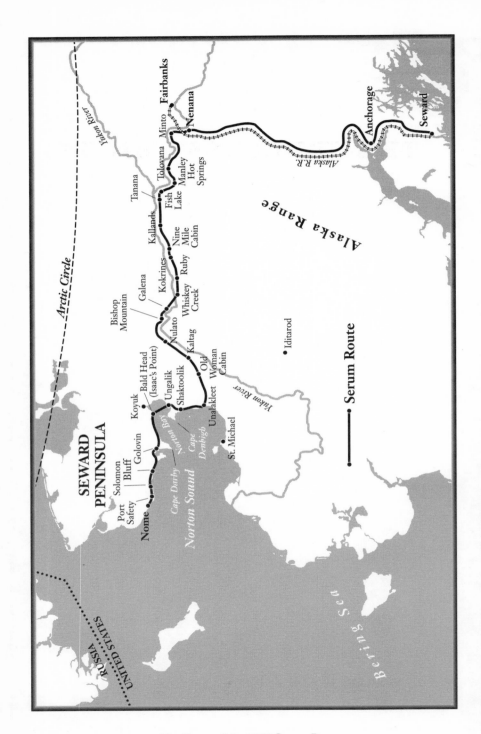

The Route of the 1925 Serum Run

THE CRUELLEST MILES

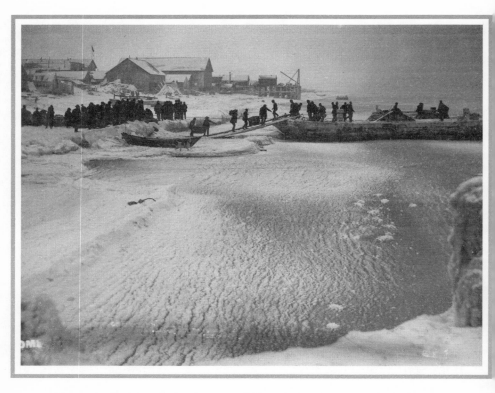

Passengers boarding the last boat out of Nome before the ice completely closes in and leaves the town icebound for seven months. (Photograph courtesy of Terrence Cole)

PROLOGUE

Icebound

"We are prisoners in a jail of ice and snow. The last boat may be justi-
fiably considered to have gone and this little community is left to its
own resources, alone with the storms, alone with the darkness and
chill of the North."

— *Nome Chronicle*

URTIS WELCH was the only doctor for hundreds of miles
along this forgotten edge of the Bering Sea, and for the past
eighteen years he had watched winter descend suddenly, as it
tends to do up in the far north. There were just two seasons here, they
said: winter and the Fourth of July. Winters were at least seven
months long in Nome, and the other seasons came and went within a
few short weeks. From July to October, the Bering Sea was free of ice
and the town was open to steamboats and schooners that sailed in
from Seattle, the closest major port, about 2,400 miles and fourteen
days away to the south. By early November, the Bering Sea would be
frozen over until the following spring and the light would be nearly
drained from the sky. The *Victoria*, usually the first passenger ship to
arrive in spring and the last to leave in the fall, would have unloaded
its cargo and headed south, leaving the town cut off from the world
save for one route: a dogsled trail that linked the town through the
Interior of Alaska to the ice-free ports in the southeast.

The unrelenting cold came on suddenly and violently, with blizzards that lasted for days and brought about an extreme isolation that
could sap the determination of the hardiest soul. Each fall, nearly half
the town's population left aboard the last ships of the season and
stayed away until spring. And yet, Welch stayed behind. He had done

so each year except once when he left on a short stint to work as a stateside doctor during the Great War. Welch had fallen for Alaska from the moment he arrived in 1907, and his fondness had grown over the years. He had once written to his sister back home in New Haven, Connecticut, that the big country provided plenty of room for him to stretch his soul.

From the time Welch was a young boy he had felt a distinct sense of otherness, and while he still found even the smallest social gesture a task—he was known to leave a dinner party when the conversation was just getting going—the boundless Alaskan space was heaven-sent. He had found himself at last, he wrote.

He was fifty now, the golden blond hair white, standing up in shocks. He looked forward to the town's annual exodus, and to his solitude.

At any time of year, Nome was a distant place, a speck on the map of America's last frontier, that vast territory of Alaska stretching out over nearly 600,000 square miles—an area as big as England, France, Italy, and Spain combined. At one end, in the southeast, were the capital, Juneau, and the territory's year-round ice-free ports. At the other end, to the northwest, was Nome. In all its parts, Alaska defied exaggeration. To the west, active volcanoes spewed smoke over a rugged North Pacific Coast, and to the east, glaciers the size of Rhode Island hovered over fjords. In the Interior, the heart of the territory, North America's tallest peak, Mount McKinley, reached up through the clouds over an endless expanse of timber. A traveler in the early 1900s said that one would have to spend a lifetime in Alaska to fully understand it, to catch the seasons' change over four climatic zones or to smell the sweet cold air as it hustled across the frozen sea. And perhaps, by the end of that lifetime, one would finally reach Nome.

In the early 1920s, Nome was the northwesternmost city in North America, a former gold rush boomtown that had lost its glitter years before. It sat 2 degrees south of the Arctic Circle on the southern shore of the Seward Peninsula, a windswept fist of land that jutted two hundred miles out into the Bering Sea. It was closer to Siberia than to any other major town in Alaska, and a little further north, on a rare, clear day in this foggy, storm-ridden world, one could see across the Bering Strait to Russia, fifty-five miles away. The international date line was a few miles off the westernmost tip of the peninsula, and one could literally see tomorrow.

From the second floor of his modest corner apartment above the Miners & Merchants Bank on Front Street, Welch and his wife, Lula, had front-row seats to the town's elaborate winter preparations. The *Victoria* was gone and the last ship of the fall season of 1924, the *Alameda*, sailed in with the town's winter supplies. It sat heavy in the water a mile and a half off the coast at the "roadstead," as near as a ship could get to shore without running aground. Nome had neither dock nor safe harbor, and the lighters and launches had to maneuver through the surf and out to the great ship before turning back to shore with their precious cargo.

On Front Street, which ran parallel to the sea, gangs of Eskimo longshoremen unloaded the cargo, which they stacked up along the waterfront and readied for storage. There were boxes of dried fruit and frozen turkeys, mountains of coal, and crates filled with butter and tea. The work went on all day and into the night. Horse carriages and wheelbarrows moved down Front Street to the hulking wooden warehouses along the shore of the Snake River on the west side of town. There was room enough to store supplies for Nome's 1,400-odd residents, as well as for many of the 10,000 other Alaskans living in scattered villages and small mining camps of the Seward Peninsula and beyond.

The town had become the region's commercial hub, and many Alaskans traveled here through the winter to buy everything from hardware to curtains and coal. If they took ill, they ended up in the care of Welch and his four nurses at Maynard Columbus Hospital, which had twenty-five beds and was considered the best-equipped medical institution in northwestern Alaska.

Front Street was never busier than in the days before the last ship sailed out. Its wooden planks creaked and its sidewalks sagged from the human traffic headed down to the waterfront. Eggs were stored in vats of brine and turkeys were laid out in cold caches built behind every home, and if the missus ran out of storage space, she could always walk down to Front Street and make a last-minute deal for a little extra room in one of the trading posts.

Children came home from the tundra with buckets filled with the last of the season's wild berries; these would be turned into preserves or better still, into cordials, which were technically illegal since Prohibition was the law of the land. Miners who had spent the summer prospecting for gold in the hills beyond Nome returned in knee-high rubber boots and woolen breeches and waited in the hotels and coffee shops to ship out. Those who stayed behind traded in their boots for warm, waterproof Native footwear called mukluks.

The U.S. Marshal was known to hand out government-issued blue tickets, which were exit visas for the insane, the destitute, and the criminally inclined. Dallying was firmly discouraged, for the *Alameda* was the only way out, and the captain could hardly risk being trapped in for the winter. The ice was the final arbiter: there was no higher authority.

Nome's permanent Eskimo population lived a mile and a half west of town on a sandbar across the mouth of the Snake River called the Sandspit, and they readied for winter as they had for centuries. Those without jobs as laborers in Nome traveled down the Bering coast with their nets to fish for a last batch of salmon or char, and the women would go to work with their curved steel knives, or *ulus*, and hang the fish up on drying racks to cure in the cold sea air. If they came upon a seal on one of their frequent trips up north, they would shoot it, load it onto their wide, skin-covered boats (umiaks), and, after a rough ride over the waves, bring it home. There it would be skinned to make mukluks and its blubber would be cut, eaten, or rendered into oil for food or fuel.

WINTER WOULD be late this year but the pace nevertheless quickened out on Front Street and along the waterfront and in the shops. Men hammered loose boards into place and lashed down the buildings, anchoring them against the wind. The Moon Springs Water Company turned off the town's only plumbing, two crude pipes running down from Anvil Creek. Holes in the wall were patched up in preparation for the blizzards, and the surfmen from the local U.S. Coast Guard station prepared to move down to the beach to haul up Nome's fleet of skiffs, schooners, and lighters.

The arctic ice pack was inching ever closer to the narrow Bering Strait and ice was forming along the shores of the Bering Sea. The sea became "an ocean of slush rolling ponderously up on the sands, crashing and splattering an icy enamel on everything it touched," said naturalist Frank Dufresne, a town resident.

On the deck of the *Alameda*, the captain knew he would have to retreat south soon or risk being crushed in the vise of the encroaching ice. It was time to batten down the crates and send out a clear message: get on board or stay behind for the winter.

As the sound of the whistle echoed across the shore, carpenters dropped their hammers, housewives paused in the street, and sled dogs roaming free on Front Street cocked their heads and, in sympathy with the *Alameda*, let out their own mournful wail.

The last lighter raced out to the ship, picked up its cargo, and returned to shore. Black smoke rose from the *Alameda*'s stacks as it built a head of steam, and the anchor went up. Finally, the bow of the ship began its slow turn southward and all of Nome took a deep breath.

They were on their own, at least until spring.

"It seemed to me that half of the people of Nome had managed to stow aboard the old steamer," said Dufresne. "I had the feeling of being deserted on an ice floe. . . . It was the worst day I ever spent in Alaska."

IN A FEW weeks, the tundra's rivers and creeks would freeze over and the frozen surface would become smooth and transparent to reflect the night stars like "tips of small torches held up from the depths." In town, hoarfrost would coat every object, and out on the Bering Sea, the waves would flatten out as the sea turned into thickening sheets of ice that might stretch as far south as the Pribilof Islands, 550 miles away.

On shore, the floes piled one on top of another in towering hummocks; a little farther north, the pressure of the sea ice had been known to force up great slabs and eject them 50 feet onto shore, crushing everything in their path. The Eskimos of the Northwest called it *ivu*—"the ice that leaps."

As the weeks passed, the sun would sink lower beneath the horizon and the fields of ice and snow would be transformed from the purest white to a wash of gold and then to a violet twilight. The days were shorter now, just four hours of sunlight, and the temperatures plunged. Finally, a cavernous silence would descend on the coast like a "great listening."

At night, as the cold hung over the land, all of Nome's wildlife and every dog and his master would hunker down. The slightest movement could puncture the arctic stillness, for the extreme cold amplified each sound. Far out at sea, one could make out the thunderclap of floes crashing into each other, and a hunter on land could hear the crunch of reindeer hooves on the crisp snow a few miles away, or the sound of a dog chewing on a bone.

Then the blizzards descended, choking gusts of snow that one resident said draws "the breath out you, then fills your nostrils and drives it back again down your throat." Another simply stated that a blizzard in Nome could feel "as if an unseen hand were clutching at my throat." One had to fight against the shrieking winds of Nome's winter storms, square one's shoulders, and lean forward with all one's weight to keep going. A short walk home through town could turn into an hour's haul and one could easily lose one's way and end up dead on the tundra behind the town.

It was as if the Great Ice Age had returned.

DR. WELCH had gone through his checklist more than once in the final days before the *Alameda* left that fall. There would have been cotton balls, ether, tongue depressors, thermometers, and medicines that needed replacing. While most of the medical supplies had arrived safely, one item was missing. Earlier that year, in the summer of 1924, Welch had noticed that the supply of diphtheria antitoxin had expired, and he had made a point of ordering up a fresh batch through the health commissioner's office in Juneau. In all of his eighteen years practicing medicine on the Seward Peninsula, he had not seen a single confirmed case of diphtheria, the deadly childhood disease. There was only the slimmest chance that he would ever need the antitoxin, yet he could never be too sure.

But now the waterfront was silent, and Welch reckoned that the order had either been ignored or misplaced. He would have to do without until next spring.

AT ABOUT the time the *Alameda* left town, an Eskimo family with four children arrived from Holy Cross, a village near the mouth of the Yukon River. The youngest child, a two-year-old, had taken ill, and when Welch examined the toddler, he found him "very much depleted and emaciated." The child refused to eat and Welch noticed that his patient had extremely foul breath. The mother told him the child had been treated for tonsillitis in Holy Cross, but the diagnosis hardly explained his weakened state. Welch questioned the parents carefully and asked whether other children in their village had tonsillitis or severe sore throats—symptoms that resembled those of diphtheria.

The parents assured him they had not.

To Welch's relief, the child's three siblings appeared healthy and robust, and he set aside his concerns: diphtheria was highly contagious, and if the siblings were infected they would have shown clear symptoms. He guessed the child might be suffering from a less severe infection.

"Many cases have come under my observation in these eighteen years that looked very suspicious, but time had always before proved that they were one of the various forms of inflammatory diseases of the throat," Welch would note in his medical records.

By the following morning, the child was dead.

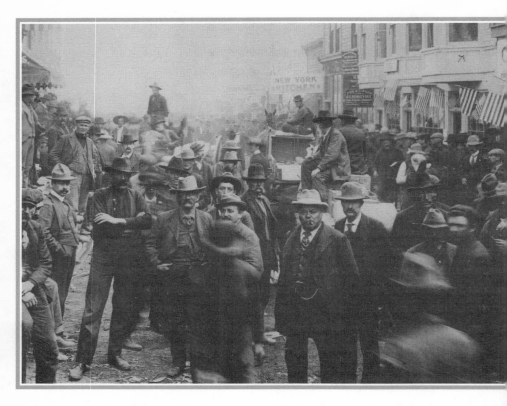

A crowd on Front Street during the heyday of gold rush Nome
in the summer of 1900. (Photograph courtesy of Terrence Cole)

1

Gold, Men, and Dogs

"Nothing in the world could have caused the building of a city where Nome is built except the thing that caused it: the finding of gold. . . . "

—Archdeacon Hudson Stuck, an Alaskan missionary

THERE WERE few worse places on earth to build a town, but Nome had gone up almost overnight after two Swedes and a Norwegian found a nugget the size of a small rock in a creek near the beach. The men came to be known as the "Three Lucky Swedes" and their discovery in 1898 would set off a stampede.

The three men had initially come to Northwest Alaska as herders for a U.S. government program designed to introduce Eskimos to reindeer as an alternative food supply. Nearly half a century of commercial whaling in the Bering Sea had devastated the Eskimos' traditional food source, which included seals and whales, and reindeer meat was thought to be a workable alternative. The youngest "Swede" was a twenty-four-year-old fisherman from the north of Norway—which at the time was run by Sweden—named Jafet Lindeberg, who had signed up for the program despite the fact that he knew almost nothing about reindeer. Lindeberg's colleagues were equally unskilled. John Brynteson got the job because he knew the reindeer program's architect, and Erik Lindblom had been a tailor in San Francisco who was said to have been shanghaied in a bar and loaded onto a whaler headed for the Bering Sea.

When the reindeer expedition was canceled, the three decided to look for gold. They had heard that there was color in the creeks of the Seward Peninsula and reckoned they had little to lose. They had about six months' prospecting experience between them, but according to one contemporary, they could barely tell "a placer from a potato patch." Either way, they knew the difference between a rock and nugget, and within weeks they were rich men. News of their good fortune spread east across Alaska into Canada and south into the United States.

NOME WAS not the first town in the far north to have sprung into life on the prospects of finding gold. In the summer of 1896, prospectors had found gold in a creek near the Klondike River, just east of the Alaskan border in Canada's Yukon Territory: the Klondike was a rich find, and newspapers and magazines ran sensational stories about the millions of dollars in placer gold discovered there. Invariably, they failed to list the perils of northern travel. Of the more than 100,000 men and women who set off from all over the world on the months-long trek, fewer than 30,000 would reach Dawson City, the boomtown that served as a gateway to the Klondike gold field.[1] Fewer still would strike it rich. Good fortune smiled more often on those with the patience or entrepreneurial skills to open up a general store or a saloon.

But gold mining was a powerful addiction. The promise of gold offered a way out of tough economic times in the United States. Years of unchecked speculation on Wall Street and faulty federal policies (one of which obligated the government to pay gold in exchange for coinable silver at values above market) had finally come to a head in 1893. Nearly fifteen thousand companies and more than six hundred banks failed, and 20 percent of the American

1. Among the tens of thousands of prospectors to the Klondike was a young writer named Jack London, who used his experiences as inspiration for writing *The Call of the Wild* (1903) and other stories.

workforce lost their jobs. Thousands of people had no savings to buy food or pay the rent. The effects of the panic were felt around the world. Thus, even with the odds stacked against them, prospectors kept coming to the Klondike. Then, in the winter of 1898, word traveled to the region that gold had been discovered on a creek on the Seward Peninsula, clear across Alaska, a distance of about eight hundred miles as the raven flies. Thousands of prospectors in the Klondike district decided to abandon their barren claims and, with picks and shovels in hand, make their way to the next shining prospect. The only route from the Klondike to Nome is along the mighty Yukon River, which stretches 2,300 miles from its headwaters in Canada across Alaska to its mouth at the Bering Sea. But by then, the Yukon River had already frozen over. The prospectors, willing by now to take just about any risk, ignored the freeze and set out by any means they could find, by dogsled or horseback, on foot, and even a few on bicycles or ice skates. The pilgrimage across Alaska's Interior to Nome was weeks long and the line stretched out for miles. It was said that the campfires along the route were seldom extinguished. "You never saw a more frenzied bunch of men impatient to get to Nome to get their crack at all this gold," said Carrie McLain, an early resident of Nome.

Several hundred miners arrived in Nome in the winter of 1898. How many didn't make it or turned back will never be known. What is clear is that those who did arrive were mostly tough and experienced trail veterans and prospectors, who were hardened by at least one far northern winter. They were known as "sourdoughs" because they often kept a supply of yeast in crocks held close to their chests. This was used to make bread on the trail and it ensured that the miner would never go hungry.

During the first winter of 1898–99, the sourdoughs settled along Anvil Creek, some five miles up from the beach where the Lucky Swedes had discovered gold. When the ice on the Bering Sea melted that summer, a new group of prospectors from the states began arriving by boat. Before long over a thousand more had set up their white tents in what was then known as the Cape Nome Mining District.[2]

The sourdoughs called the new arrivals "cheechakoes," a combination of Native Indian words meaning "newcomer." The new boys brought a dangerous element to the mix: they were, for the most part, naive. Few of them had ever been this far north; they had only the slightest notion of the harshness and isolation they would face once winter came and the Bering Sea froze; and their food and fuel would soon run out. Nome's establishment considered the newcomers a threat and worried that the town was in for a rough time. Everyone knew that more prospectors would be coming.

Early that summer, an aging Idaho prospector named John Hummel, too sick to hike up to Anvil Creek to hunt for gold, had decided to try out his luck on the beach. He talked a younger man into doing the physical work for him, and soon the beach was yielding $100 a day. The news went out that Nome's beaches were made of gold and that there were enough nuggets for anyone who could bend down and pick one up. Gold, they said, came in with the tide. But by the time word of Hummel's luck had reached the states late in the fall of 1899, the Bering Sea was frozen over and winter had set in. There was no way to reach Nome until the following year. Through the

2. When the miners registered the town with the U.S. Post Office to receive mail, they initially named the mining district Anvil City after a nearby rock that looked like the blacksmith's tool. The postal authorities, however, rejected the name because another Alaskan mining camp had already claimed the title, and so instead the boomtown was called Nome, after the cape of the same name thirteen miles to the east. The naming of Cape Nome is widely believed to have been the result of a cartographer's bad handwriting. A draftsman aboard HMS *Herald*, which was in search of the missing crew of the 1845 Franklin Expedition, had apparently written "? Name" on his map when the ship passed by a cape on the Seward Peninsula that had not been marked. When the map was later drawn in permanent pen, the cartographer mistook the question mark for a C and "Name" for "Nome." Some locals in Nome believe in another version. The Eskimo expression *kn-no-me* means "I don't know" and is thought to have been the answer Natives gave when foreign visitors landing on the shore asked the likely question, "What's the name of this place?"

winter, the legend spread from one port city to the next, across the United States and beyond its borders, and thousands of would-be entrepreneurs began to prepare for the trek up the Pacific Northwest for their summer assault on Nome in 1900.

Reports of the new diggings on the edge of the Bering Sea reached the governor of Alaska as well: one of the miners had made it his business to travel by boat and trail to warn Governor John G. Brady that mayhem and lawlessness threatened the new camp. They needed help. Brady contacted federal officials and requested that troops be sent in to uphold the law. "These men are mad with the lust for gold," Brady reportedly said upon hearing the news. "Conditions will be desperate unless a restraining influence can be exerted. . . . You can hardly imagine to what depths a mining camp, shut away from civilization for eight months by a thousand miles of impassable ice, may descend. . . ."

By the summer of 1900, as the ice melted out on the Bering Sea, more than fifty ships were waiting off the coast of Nome. It was a ragged armada of steamers and ungainly paddlewheels, some more seaworthy than others. On board were thousands of would-be prospectors who had come straight from San Francisco and Seattle and others from St. Michael, the deepwater port nearest to the mouth of the Yukon River, where they had been stranded en route from other small mining camps in Alaska and the Yukon Territory.

The journey had been difficult enough: many of the prospectors had had to wait in one of the harbors of the Aleutian Chain until the ice melted and the boats could pass through to the Bering Sea. After weeks on board, they were anxious to step out onto the gold-rich beaches and try their luck; but first they had to disembark. In the heaving surf, passengers with bags and cargo scaled down the towering steamship decks to the lighters below. The boats banged against the hulls, rising and falling to the rhythm of the sea, and after everyone had piled on, the lighters were hauled to shore with heavy ropes.

For those who had risked everything to come this far, to turn back empty-handed would mean a return to a life of certain poverty, with the added sting of ridicule. They fell onto the beach with picks and shovels and immediately went to work. According to one account, one desperate miner dropped to his hands and knees when he came upon shore: there was not a single nugget in sight. Grief-stricken, he cried out, "It's all a lie!" Then he shot himself in the head.

Geologists would later discover that there had been only a limited supply of "Hummel's Gold" on the beach, trace deposits left in the sand by eons of erosion. Furthermore, the miners had been facing the wrong way: the real gold lay on the tundra behind them, in the creeks and rivers outside of town.

More than twenty thousand cheechakoes arrived that summer of 1900, and they propped up their white camp tents along the beach. The tents stretched out for thirty miles along the coast. "It seemed as if a great albatross had settled on the shore," one eyewitness said. "Its wings—the white tents of the busy gold seekers—stretching up and down the coast; its gray-breast the huddled group of stores and cabins hastily constructed of driftwood."

There was no need to register a claim, for the beach was considered public property, and no sooner had anyone landed than they threw down their tools and set to work in the sand. There were Norwegians and Frenchmen, Russians and Americans, a babel of languages above the pounding of the surf. Along the shore, a line of wooden rockers stood like a phalanx of defensive artillery. The tall, unsteady devices had a narrow rectangular sluice box lined with copper plating and quicksilver to catch the gold. There were other, more elaborate mechanical contraptions with wheels, engines, and pulleys. The sound could be deafening: the jerry-built machines clanged and coughed and the miners shook their rockers as the water pushed through in a cascade of gravel and sand. The surf boomed.

On Front Street, above the beach, they built gambling halls and saloons from the cords of lumber, windows, and tools hauled in from the states. There was scant consideration given to the tides, and many of the buildings were set dangerously close to the edge of the sea, just yards away from the driftwood and jetsam. The builders would eventually regret their haste and imprudence.

By the end of summer the town had risen on the tundra. There were sixteen law offices open for business along Front Street, as well as twelve general stores, four real estate offices, an equal number of drugstores, five laundries, four bathhouses, three fruit and cigar stores, as many watchmakers, and a masseuse. One section of the street called the "stockade" was for the bordellos. This was the first stop for the miners who came up from the beach or hiked down from the creeks. The prostitutes lived behind Front Street in rowhouses no better than shacks. "Hoo-Hoo" Henderson, one of the most popular, knew every trick in the book and earned her sobriquet by shouting, "Hoo-Hoo! Hoo-Hoo!" whenever she faked orgasm.

The gunslinger Wyatt Earp, a legend after his gunfight at the O.K. Corral, moved up to Nome and became co-owner of Dexter's Saloon, the first two-story building in town. Dexter's had a bar downstairs and more than twelve rooms for rent upstairs. The western writer Rex Beach lived here and filled his notebooks with tales of Nome. His book *The Spoilers*, based on the story of a corrupt federal judge involved in a conspiracy to steal claims, became a best-seller. Tex Rickard started his career staging boxing matches for Nome's miners, then moved on to New York and built Madison Square Garden, becoming one of the first great sports impresarios.

The town sat just 150 miles south of the Arctic Circle, and the sun stayed up for twenty hours and the drinking and brawling went on forever in the sixty-odd bars that sprang up. Player pianos were kept oiled, the dancehall girls charged a dollar a twirl to shuffle across roughhewn boards, and there was enough money and time to go around forever—or so it seemed.

Coal sold for $100 a ton, eggs were $4 a dozen, and miners doled out pokes of gold dust without a second thought. Gold dust was used as money because there was not enough currency in circulation. Bars, hotels, and stores had weights and scales to measure out the gold, sometimes honestly and sometimes not. One weigher claimed he would use syrup as hair tonic so that when he weighed out the gold with slightly damp fingers and ran his fingers through his hair, he had a sizable stash at the end of each day. Within weeks, many of the miners had gone bust and ended up destitute on the beach. Crime was up: on the creeks, miners armed with guns and knives jumped claims; down on the beach, thieves would creep up to the tents and lower chloroform-drenched rags through the flaps and onto the mouths of sleeping miners. Then they would grab the gold and vanish. "The greed of man went farther here than in any other place I have ever known," one hardened miner recalled.

Governor Brady's federal soldiers managed to establish some semblance of peace, but they found themselves overwhelmed by the sheer numbers in Nome or by the lure of gold. Half of them deserted and fled up the creeks with panning trays. One enlisted man was so concerned by what he had seen that he returned to the states to warn others. "To those who contemplate going to Alaska, to battle with the climate, to cross almost impassable country, to ford streams nearly as cold in the summer as they are during the long Arctic winters, I would say 'don't,' " said Lieutenant H. French.

Nome was well on the road to perdition when, on the afternoon of September 12, 1900, a strong gale blew in from the south with 70-mile-an-hour winds and lifted up the sea. Massive waves fell on shore and battered the town for twenty-four hours. Prospectors who had stayed behind in their tents were said to have been swept out to sea, and as the ocean rose, the waves crashed all the way up to Front Street and beyond. The storm splintered buildings and hurled lighters and boats onto the street, smashing whatever was in the way. Shards of glass, wood, and metal sailed through the air, mining contraptions tumbled over, and a number of ships were sunk.

As the storm died down, a crowd of townspeople lined up along the beach in silence and watched as a phantom ship drifted toward shore in full sail. It was the triple-masted schooner *Sequoia*, believed to have been lost at sea years earlier. The ship had been another victim of the Bering Sea, the graveyard of the Pacific, and it brought with it an ominous message: Nome would be no easy ride.

As the waves receded and debris piled up on the shore, thousands of prospectors who had survived months of lawlessness, drunkenness, and poverty decided they'd had enough. They stood quietly in long lines on the beach and waited for the next ship out. They were called the "cold feets," and they all had one thing in common: they could no longer bear the thought of another day in Nome.

By late October, most of the twenty thousand men and women who had arrived a few months earlier had shipped out. Someone would later comment that "even God leaves on the last boat" out of Nome. This would bear repeating every fall.

The storm marked the end of the rush to Nome. As far as the rest of the world was concerned, the town had up and vanished from the headlines and no longer existed.

But as the last boat left in October 1900, roughly five thousand miners chose to stay and build up from the ruins. Some had fallen in love with the north, others had taken a shine to the unpretentious ways of Alaskan society. Others simply had nowhere else to go.

THE KLONDIKE and Nome stampedes transformed Alaska. With the near doubling of Alaska's population between 1890 and 1900, new trails were cleared and existing ones widened and improved. The federal government set up military posts in Nome and St. Michael as well as in the Interior, where new mining camps and towns had sprung up, and soldiers strung up telegraph wires so the forts and towns could communicate with each other and with the states. By 1903, Nome had become part of an impressive telegraph system operated by the U.S. Army Signal Corps, and the territory's overwhelming isolation was significantly reduced.[3] In addition, the federal

---

3. Messages from Nome to the states went over three handlings: radio, telegraph, and submarine cable. The U.S. Signal Corps made several attempts to link Nome via a submarine cable across Norton Sound to St. Michael, but the constant shifting of the ice across the seabed floor repeatedly carried the cable out to sea. With no other option available, the Corps turned to the relatively new technology of "wireless telegraphy"; it built 200-foot towers at each end of Norton Sound, 133 miles apart, and successfully made Nome a part of the system. The radio link, however, was not without its own temporary problems. A blizzard in 1904 tore the roof off the station on the Nome side, filling the room up with snow and killing the fire in the potbelly stove that kept the operators warm. In a matter of seconds the temperature inside the station dropped to nearly 70 below and the water in the 6-horsepower gasoline engine that ran the generator froze, cracking the cylinder.

government established a mail delivery service, which in winter relied upon dog teams. One route ran all the way northwest to Nome.

The arrival of the mail team was among the most exciting events to watch in Nome. It was not uncommon for the driver to have twenty-five dogs pulling two sleds with a 1,500-pound load, and when they arrived they were snubbed down securely to a telephone pole before a crowd in front of the post office. No other draft animal was more suited for travel in the north, and in Nome, as well as in much of Alaska, "if you didn't own a dog team, or if you didn't have a lot of money, you walked," as one Alaskan U.S. Deputy Marshal, Bert Hansen, put it. From the beginning, Nome depended on its dogs. Teams were drafted into service as mail trucks, ambulances, freight trains, and long-distance taxis. The demand for sled dogs was so high, particularly during the northern gold rushes, that the supply of dogs ran out and a black market for the animals sprang up in the states. Any dog that looked as if it could pull a sled or carry a saddlebag— whether or not it was suited to withstand the cold—was kidnapped and sold in the north. "It was said at the time that no dog larger than a spaniel was considered safe on the streets" of West Coast port towns, said one sled dog historian.

Drivers liked to work with large dogs because they often carried loads one and a half times heavier than their teams. Newfoundlands, St. Bernards, and hounds were popular imports, and they were crossbred with the indigenous dog population. In Nome, the imports were bred with malamutes, named after the Eskimo Mahlemuit people. Over the past several hundred years, the Eskimos had used and bred their dogs to freight heavy loads for relatively short distances. When miners crossbred the Native dogs with Newfoundlands and St. Bernards, the outcome was sometimes astonishing: mutts that weighed as much as 125 pounds. The malamute nearly disappeared, yet its name lived on; miners in Nome as well as in the Interior often called their mixed-bred dogs malamutes.

Alaska's most skillful drivers and trainers were well known throughout the territory. Nome resident Scotty Allan acquired a reputation early on for being able to subdue even the most reprobate of canines and transform them into hardworking, loyal sled dogs. With his soft Scottish accent and patient temperament, he could "gentle anything on four legs."

Putting together a team took time and skill: dogs did not come in teams and each member was selected for its relative speed, strength, and gait so that it would match the other dogs in the string. The animals were taught directional commands and to move and think in unison. Each had its own personality, and it was not always easy to bring them in line.

Generally, the teams were set up in pairs on either side of the main line, or gang line, attached to the front of the sled. The dog in front (sometimes there were two) was called the leader and was the smartest of the team. Behind the leader were several pairs of "swing dogs" and closest to the sled were the "wheel dogs," the biggest and strongest of the team. Sleds were generally between 9 and 14 feet in length and made of hickory or birchwood. They were lashed together with rawhide for greater flexibility and had a curved piece in front called a brush bow that acted like a bumper and protected the sled against shrubs or trees. If the driver, who stood on runners extending out from the back, was carrying a particularly heavy load or driving uphill, he could help the dogs along by pedaling with one leg as if he were on a scooter or push from behind at a jog.

On the Alaskan trail, the sled dogs became partners in a game of survival. Drivers depended on their dogs so that they could make a living as freighters, mailmen, and trappers, and relied on the animals' skill and intelligence to get them safely across the rough, dangerous terrain. In return for their labor, the dogs required care and protection.

The majority of the residents in Nome owned their own team, and the dogs seemed to rule the streets. At one point dogs became such a hazard that the town passed a law requiring them to wear bells. There were more dogs than people and their howls, known as "the malamute chorus," could always be heard throughout the night. The dogs of Nome were almost as important as the citizens. Many roamed free when they were not working and some accompanied their masters into the saloons. An attorney named Albert Fink, who years later would defend Al Capone, would tip his hat whenever he passed a husky he particularly respected, and he once managed to persuade a jury that his sled dog Peg was acting in self-defense when he slaughtered twenty-eight sheep owned by the Pacific Cold Storage Company.

"Is Alaska a dog country or a sheep country?" he asked the jury. "Look at my star wheeler—look at Peg—look at that ear mangled by murderous mutton—look at his eyes, his noble head. Gentlemen—choose."

The jury found the dog's owner innocent and in their verdict explained that in Nome, sheep had to look out for themselves: "This aims to be a dog country."

Owners bragged endlessly about their teams and detailed the courage and skill of their lead dogs. They would fight anyone who dared to criticize their faithful companions, and they bet on who had the strongest, fastest, and smartest animal. In the saloons of this newly decorous town, it was not uncommon for fists to fly over such claims.

IN THE fall of 1907, around the wood-burning stove at the Board of Trade Saloon, Albert Fink, Scotty Allan, and a few friends established the Nome Kennel Club with the intention of organizing a dogsled race. Over the next several weeks, Fink and his colleagues devised a long-distance race like no other. The 408-mile, round-trip trek through every imaginable terrain would test the mettle, intelligence, and endurance of dog and driver. The route ran between the ice hummocks of the Bering Sea, up mountains, over the tundra, and through a blizzard-swept chute called Death Valley. It followed the telegraph lines linking the mining villages on the Seward Peninsula, and would thus allow gamblers and enthusiasts to track the race from the relative safety of the town's saloons. For the first fifty miles, the trail ran east along the blustery coast and up Topkok Mountain, a steep, 600-foot incline rising up over the sea. It turned inland and climbed steadily through willow and cottonwood bush, then across creeks and rivers to

Council, a mining settlement eighty miles from Nome. The route snaked through valleys, tiptoed along ridge tops as narrow as a sled was wide, and sloped off in half-mile-long drops. Then, about 120 miles into the race, the trail entered Death Valley.

If the musher had survived this far, he climbed a glacier to cross over the Continental Divide—the boundary line separating the Pacific and Arctic Ocean watersheds. Thirty miles farther lay the turnaround mark, the village of Candle, which was situated near Kotzebue Sound on the north shore of the peninsula. An exhausted and sleep-deprived driver would have to turn around and face the same terrible 204 miles all over again.

Officials called it the All Alaska Sweepstakes. Others called it "reckless." The inhabitants of Nome, however, welcomed the race with enthusiasm. They were tired of the deadly dullness of the seven-month-long winter, and donated time and money to preparations for the first race. It took place in April 1908 and was such a success that it became an annual event until 1917, when World War I intervened, severely disrupting Alaska's economy.

The All Alaska Sweepstakes transformed the isolated town. By the start of each race every April, Nome became a frenzied festival. Miners from the Seward Peninsula came down and every dog team owner dreamed of winning the thousands of dollars in prize money. (The first year the prize was $10,000.) Year after year, news of the event was covered widely across Alaska and in the states, and Nome, now "Dog Capital of the World," was once again in the headlines. There was no other race like it at the time—as the official race pamphlet said, it "easily towers above all other contests of physical endurance, for both man and beast."

Bunting and brightly colored pennants representing the colors of each team hung across the street, and the gold and yellow flags of the Kennel Club snapped in the breeze at the starting line at Barracks Square. Storekeepers hung signs reading GONE TO THE DOGS on their doorknobs, and the gamblers and spectators were out in force. At race time, they would crowd close to the line and invariably delay the start. Bartenders dressed in white waistcoats left their jobs to catch a glimpse, and those who could not squeeze through the crowds climbed up the telephone poles and onto rooftops for a better view.

As the race began, the crowds rushed to the saloons. The Board of Trade became race headquarters and was usually the most crowded. Here, the names of the drivers were listed on a large rectangular chalkboard across the room from the mahogany bar, next to paintings of nude drunken revelers.

As the drivers passed each telegraph station on the course, the "Information Kid" would record the changing positions and times and the gamblers would press up close to decipher his scrawl. The books stayed open nearly until the end of the four-day race, the odds shifting as quickly as the gamblers could buy drinks. It was chaos: one spectator said it was less like gambling and "more like dealing on the stock exchange."

In the first years of the sweepstakes, Scotty Allan won most of the races, and for years his team were considered Alaska's top dogs. Allan had a natural gift with animals and had trained horses and dogs since he was a twelve-year-old in Scotland. To prepare for the sweepstakes, he experimented with the dogs' diets and spent hours in the kennels examining the paws of each dog, trimming the claws so that they would not catch in the snow, and greasing between the pads. He made rabbit-fur covers for his team, which had shorter hair than most of the local dogs, and designed booties for their feet, which were more tender and prone to injury. He designed racing harnesses that were lighter and less cumbersome and made the traditional freight sled lighter and he replaced its handlebars with a crossbar that made it easier to push. His basic designs are still in use today.

By late 1915, word of Allan's reputation for handling sled dogs had reached the French army, which turned to him for help in the war against Germany. Supply lines to army units in eastern France had become hindered by deep snow and the French had heard that the sled dogs of Nome could succeed where horses and mules had failed. Allan needed more than four hundred sled dogs for this secret mission. To avoid skyrocketing prices, he went around Nome and its surrounding villages and quietly bought up 106 dogs, and harnesses and sleds, as well as 2 tons of dried salmon for food.

To transport the animals, he rigged up a 300-foot towline and attached the dogs in pairs to the heavy rope. The end of the towline was hooked to two draft horses and a heavy carriage that held the dogs back in case they got too excited or tried to flee. A crowd watched as Allan drove the team up a bobbing gangplank to a barge and then out to a ship waiting offshore. They sailed to Canada, where they boarded a guarded train and traveled to Quebec; there Allan assembled over 300 more dogs from the Canadian Arctic, 60 sleds, and 350 harnesses. Then Allan and his "K9 Corps" sailed to France on the *Pomeranian*, an old cargo ship that had recently been brought out of retirement.

Once on shore, Allan divided the dogs into sixty teams and trained fifty cavalrymen to drive them. They hauled 90 tons of ammunition to a stranded unit in the Vosges Mountains, and helped soldiers lay down communication lines to a detachment that had been cut off by the Germans. In addition, they hauled in the wounded to field hospitals. "It was enough to make one forget all about the war, even when the shells were singing, to see a line half a mile long of dog teams tearing down the mountain to the base depot, every blue devil whooping and yelling and trying to pass the one ahead," Allan remembered.

THE REPUTATION of the sweepstakes also helped to turn Nome into a magnet for explorers and adventurers who needed dogs and guides for northern expeditions, and the town became a way station for crews en route to the Arctic's upper reaches. It was also the last chance for explorers to outfit their crews with sturdy equipment, men, dogs, and fur clothes. Most of the residents and visitors to Nome relied heavily upon the local Eskimo community. Apart from working menial jobs for the town's mining companies and other concerns, they manufactured the large majority of clothes, harnesses, and sleds. In 1905, a missionary had set up a cooperative behind St.

Joseph's Church where the Eskimos could make fur parkas and sled-ding equipment with traditional tools. These were sold to the locals and to arctic explorers who passed through the town, including Vilh-jalmur Stefansson and Roald Amundsen.

Demand for Eskimo clothes supported two separate populations of craftsmen. Each summer, the Eskimos from the rocky King Islands arrived on the east side of town to sew garments and carve ivory curios such as cribbage boards and miniature dog teams. Even the more sedentary residents preferred the Native fur parkas and boots to their own wool and leather clothes. By 1908, the high school's white basketball team was wearing uniforms consisting of short Native parkas with intricate designs. The Eskimos' influence was wide-spread: during celebrations such as the Fourth of July, Native games competed with the brass bands and parades; there were kayak races in the Snake River and a blanket toss on the tundra, in which a huge swath of walrus skin was sewn together and held taut while a contest-ant was hurled into the air. Traditionally, Natives used the blanket toss as a tool for spotting whales.

Gradually, Eskimos integrated into Nome's community, where interracial marriages were not uncommon. Yet, under federal law, Natives went to separate schools and some residents recalled Natives sitting in their own section in the town's only moviehouse, the Dream Theatre, or occupying their own side of the church for Sunday mass.

WITH THE end of the All Alaska Sweepstakes and the coming of World War I, Nome settled into a quiet routine. By 1925, the popu-lation was significantly lower than in the years after the first of the cold feets had fled. There had been storms and fires, and the war had led to an inflation that tripled the cost of mining. Many operations throughout Alaska went out of business. Since about 60 percent of Alaskan society was dependent upon the industry in one way or another, thousands of people throughout the territory migrated south. Nome was no exception. The town's population was reduced to 975 whites and 455 Eskimos or interracial residents.

The glamour of the gold rush days and the excitement of the sweepstakes era were gone and many of the buildings were vacant or decaying. It was still possible to make out a faded advertisement for a lawyer or a saloon left over from the gold rush. Whenever a resident spoke about the good old days to a newcomer, the "places seemed to straighten up on their old foundations and come alive with history." Tony Polet, Nome's grocer, built his kitchen and living room in what had once been the Discovery Saloon. There were abandoned miners' cabins still equipped with their barrel stoves, and one could still find a pair of trousers and a jacket hanging on the wall, as if a miner had stepped out for a moment. Mining equipment sat rusting on the tundra and along the beach, and nothing was thrown out. You never knew when you might have use for the wood or the metal. Gold remained a principal industry in Nome, but now it was controlled by Hammon Consolidated Gold Fields, a conglomerate from the states. The company had bought up all the claims and water ditches of Pioneer Mining Company, the firm that had been started by the Lucky Swedes.

Before Hammon's arrival, Pioneer miners used jets of pressurized water to blast away gold-laden gravel banks and wash the material through giant wooden sluice boxes that separated the gold from the silt. Hammon spent good money to upgrade the equipment, and miners now worked with huge, electric-powered dredges that sat like houseboats out in ponds in the gold fields. A conveyor belt of buckets dug up the thawed earth while a chute spat out a steady stream of stones, gravel, and dirt. The dredges were mobile and moved slowly and destructively across the tundra, taking the ponds with them as they filled in the water behind them with tailings from the chute. Inside the housing, the gold was separated by revolving screens and captured by sluices that ran alongside the machine.

To one first-time visitor from the states arriving in the 1920s, the town looked "like last year's bird nest." But from a purely Alaskan perspective, Nome was a smart and bustling outpost. Lula Welch, arriving with her husband, Dr. Welch, in 1919 from the Candle mining camp on the northern side of Seward Peninsula, felt an immediate charge of excitement.

"It was so big and bright, I felt it must be New York City," she said.

It was the first time in twelve years that the Welches had seen an electric light. The Welches first landed in northwestern Alaska in 1907, disembarking from the *Victoria* at Nome. They headed straight for the rough, inland mining camp of Council, where Welch had bought a private practice from a friend just months after the clinic he and Lula ran in Oakland was destroyed by the San Francisco earthquake. They had intended to stay for only a year, but they remained in Council for eight years. Welch worked with a portable operating table in a three-bed ward about 20 feet long and lit by a kerosene lamp. "If there happened to be a patient in the ward he could watch the operation or turn over and look the other way," he wrote in a brief memoir. In 1915, the couple moved to Candle, an outpost even more remote and primitive. Nome felt like a luxurious new beginning for them. It had its own weekly newspaper, the *Nome Nugget*, bakeries, two restaurants, social halls, a library, a U.S. Marshal's office, and the Dream Theatre, "a hall as run-down as its old movies of the pre-1920 days."

There was a jeweler and a dressmaker. One could join social and literary groups and take singing and dancing lessons. Nome took itself seriously as the region's commercial center and laid its streets out in a grid, adding to the air of importance. For a place so very handicapped by its location, there was a remarkable array of services available.

In winter, Ed the Scavenger Man picked up the garbage and carted it out to the town dump, which was marked by a line of red flags along the frozen Bering Sea. "Honey buckets" placed beneath the outhouses were picked up and replaced. If a resident needed water, he put out a green cardboard "W" sign in his front window and his 5-gallon drum would be filled. In summer, water was piped down from the natural springs outside town.

Despite the ramshackle surroundings, Nome's residents managed to maintain a sort of windswept cosmopolitanism. Strangers and misfits mixed easily. The children took singing lessons and their parents put on plays and dances at Eagle Hall and the Arctic Brotherhood Hall. It was like living on an island, a close-knit community whose very architecture seemed designed for intimacy. The houses were built about two-thirds normal size to save on heat and building costs. What they lacked in space, they made up for in intricate woodwork. The homes had arched doorways, detailed moldings, cornices, fancy staircases, and wainscoting.

Still, life was hard enough. Mining remained a cold, wet profession, and dog driving was exhausting and dangerous and required weeks away from home. The wives and children often had to help out with the family finances. Some wives cooked in the canteens run by Hammon or did laundry for a restaurant or one of the wealthier families. Children also did chores around the house or took odd jobs. Joe Walsh, whose father was a miner, added to the family income by selling fresh milk from a sled pulled by his dog, Turk. Walsh owned the only two cows in town. They were hard to keep in the cold, so Walsh visited them every night in the abandoned miners' cabin he had turned into a stall and made sure they had enough blankets.

Nome relied on a spirit of cooperation and good citizenship, a surprising transformation in light of the town's recent and sordid history. It seemed as if every citizen had an unofficial duty, and each took it very seriously. The trails were maintained in part by volunteers who made sure wooden stakes marking the route were kept in place, and the widow Rattenburg, who worked as a seamstress and dressmaker, sewed the red cotton pennants that marked the trail for miners heading out to Hammon's dredging sites. Shopkeepers kept their stoves well stoked in case a traveler needed to warm up, and Dr. Welch treated his patients whether or not they could afford to pay.

Over the years, several people had wandered out into the tundra and frozen to death, so the town fathers built an eight-foot electric cross on the steeple of St. Joseph's Church to serve as a beacon for lost travelers.

It still remained an inauspicious place to build a town. One would be hard-pressed to find a single foot of arable soil or a tree for protection against wind and sun. Burying the dead was hard work: beneath a foot of topsoil was permafrost that never thawed. It would take hours to dig a shallow grave, and the bodies sometimes drifted into town, washed up by the seasonal floods. And yet, aside from the exigencies of its location, Nome functioned much like any other American community of the 1920s. There were contentious school board meetings and internecine civic squabbles of one sort or another.

Nome's residents knew exactly how much coal to order and how many turkeys, cans of evaporated milk, eggs, and medical supplies they needed for winter. They knew how to plug up their keyholes to protect against blizzards and how to reach the doctor or hospital if their children became ill. But they enjoyed a false sense of security, for the town's isolation could quickly turn an average crisis into a catastrophe. If the weather turned suddenly, or there was a fire, or if a cargo ship sank, they might as well be on the dark side of the moon.

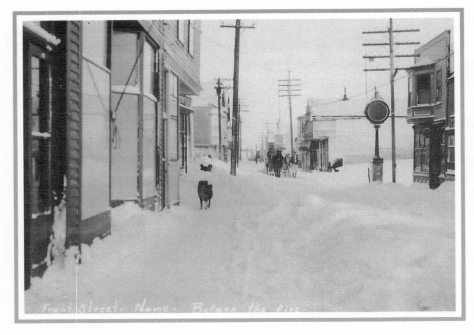

Front Street nearly abandoned upon news of the outbreak. (Authors' collection)

2

Outbreak

"All by ourselves. The last boat has gone and we are, to use the homely phrase, 'alone with ourselves.' . . ."

—Nome Nugget

D R. WELCH remembered each year according to whom he'd treated and how they'd fared: some memories were stronger than others, and some years stood out. One summer there was an infection attributed to mosquitoes; another year there were a number of minor injuries out at the mining camps.

He remembered Bobby Brown fairly clearly. It was 1917 and at the time Welch was living in Candle. Brown had been raced in from a mill by dogsled with internal bleeding and one leg nearly severed at the muscle. He had been mangled in the course of his work, and Welch managed to keep him alive long enough to see his family one last time.

No doctor could forget the 1918–19 influenza pandemic, though Welch should have been thankful he had seen only the tail end of it in Nome. He had felt useless as a physician and was unable to keep many from dying.

This year, ever since the *Alameda* sailed off, there had been one tonsillitis case after another, including the strange case of the young Eskimo child from Holy Cross. And just this morning, December 24, Welch had another sick child on his hands. She was a seven-year-old Eskimo Norwegian girl named Margaret Solvey Eide, who had a severe sore throat and a slight fever.

Welch thought she might be suffering from follicular tonsillitis, but her mother, perhaps guided by her Native superstition, wouldn't let him examine her. Her husband had gone Outside—beyond the territory—on a business trip.

Welch told the girl to stay in bed for the holidays and rest up, and afterwards he walked home through town. For weeks, the shop windows along Front Street had been filled with skates and sleds, dolls and Erector sets for Christmas.

But Welch wasn't feeling much of a holiday spirit. There had been so many children suffering from colds, and he had been out on so many house calls that no man in his situation could have been in high spirits or had much energy. Then again, it was no secret that Welch was a complicated man, who often traveled under a cloud.

Other residents were in a jollier mood. It was, after all, a special time of year, and in the mid-1920s the highlight was Christmas Eve at Eagle Hall. Every year, many of the town's two hundred children filed into the cavernous wooden structure which had served, during the town's boom days, as a venue for minstrel shows and boxing matches. Nome tried its best to celebrate the holiday in the traditional way, trees and all, which was no mean feat given the fact that the nearest evergreen was ninety miles away—at least a two-day trip—to the southeast near the village of White Mountain. The trees may have seemed stunted to an outsider, but to the children and parents of Nome, who were used to the low-scrub views of the tundra, the White Mountain evergreens seemed huge. Nome's volunteers headed out on their dogsleds with axes and saws: they brought back a little tree for the hospital, another for the school, and a third for Barracks Square. The best was reserved for the Community Christmas Eve celebration at Eagle Hall.

Set up center stage, the Christmas tree was "asparkle with tinsel, aglow with lights," and red and green crepe paper billowed down from the balcony. The fireplace crackled; there was hoarfrost on the windows and stockings hung from the mantel bulging with Cracker Jacks, candy canes, pencils, and fresh oranges and apples, delicacies which had arrived on the last ship in the fall and were set aside for the holiday.

The choir from the Eskimo church came down the aisle with

candles in hand and sang carols in their native tongue, and the other children came out on stage and reenacted the story of Christmas. Toward the end, they could hear the faintest jingle of sleigh bells outside, and soon the heavy double doors of Eagle Hall swung open and there was Fire Chief Conrad Yenney in his Santa suit, driving a black cutter sleigh pulled along by two skittish reindeer wearing red and green pom-poms and silver bells. The animals bucked and strained and had to be held in check by a handler, while Yenney leapt off the sleigh, bounded up to the stage, and handed out the stockings. When he was done, he drove back out into the night. Coffee and cake were served and "the whole town was alive, gossiping and carrying on."

When the bells of St. Joseph's Church rang out at midnight, they all walked to the service through the newly fallen snow, and when it was over, they headed home along Front Street and Steadman Avenue. The streets stretched out before them in drifts of snow that had been hardened by the wind and constant traffic of dogsleds and mukluks. Some of the drifts were as high as the second-story apartments above the shops.

At home, the turkeys, which had been thawed out and soaked for hours in soda water and salt before being roasted, were devoured. Tomorrow, Nome would become a giant playground.

In the days that followed, between Christmas and New Year's, they would play the games they always played during winter. They would put on their double-runner ice skates and go out on the Snake River and Bering Sea or slide down the steep banks of Front Street on their sleds and mukluks. Jean Summers-Wolf, the daughter of the superintendent of Hammon Consolidated Gold Fields, would always remember a game of "crack the whip" which ended with her sailing out over the ice for what seemed forever and landing unhurt in an Eskimo fishing hole.

But one little girl missed the festivities that year. Margaret Eide's condition deteriorated as the days passed, and on December 28 Welch received notice that the young girl had died. Welch asked her mother if he could perform an autopsy, but again she refused to let him examine the body. The case bothered him. "Death from tonsillitis is rare, but nevertheless sometimes does occur," he wrote.

The holiday season continued. The Rebekehas Women's Group held their annual New Year's Eve party for all the children in Nome at the Odd Fellows Hall and Hazel Modini's folks capped off the season by throwing a party for their daughter's fifth birthday, events all duly reported in the *Nome Nugget*.

By January 1925, there was more disturbing news: two other Native children out on the Sandspit had reportedly died. Welch began to suspect the worst.

Then, on the afternoon of Tuesday, January 20, it all came to a head. As he was making his rounds at Maynard Columbus, Welch checked in on a three-year-old boy named Billy Barnett whom he had admitted almost two weeks ago after the boy developed a sore throat, swollen glands, fever, and fatigue. Within days of entering the hospital, Billy had presented a disturbing new symptom: thick grayish lesions in his throat and nasal membranes.

The gray and bloody ulcers on Billy's tonsils and in his mouth cavity were characteristic of an ancient and dreaded bacteria, a centuries-old killer of young children which, for good reason, was often referred to as "the strangler." Its official name is diphtheria.

Diphtheria is an airborne bacteria that thrives in the moist membranes of the throat and nose and releases a powerful toxin that makes its victims tired and apathetic. In two to five days, other, more deadly symptoms would appear: a slight fever and red ulcers at the back of the throat and in the mouth. As the bacteria multiplied and more toxin was released, the ulcers thickened and expanded, forming a tough, crusty, almost leathery membrane made up of dead cells, blood clots, and dead skin. The membrane colonized ever larger portions of the mouth and the throat, until it had nowhere left to go and advanced down the windpipe, slowly suffocating the victim.

It was a slow, painful, and frightening way to die. The majority of victims were young children between the ages of one and ten years, and the "anxious, struggling, pitiful expression of impending suffocation" in child after child infected during one epidemic, as a doctor described it, deeply affected physicians.

"The most distressing pictures covering the walls of the memory chamber of my brain," a nineteenth-century physician wrote in the aftermath of an epidemic in a Michigan village that had manifested "every possible complication and sequel" of the disease. Before the advent of antitoxin at the turn of the century, doctors could offer little comfort but their presence and prayers.

But antitoxin, which was made from the serum of immunized horses, did cure the disease. The problem was that Welch had only a limited supply and it was old. He was concerned that the antitoxin had become unstable over time, and since the golden rule of any doctor is to avoid harming the patient, Welch decided not to inject Billy.[1] There was still a slim chance in his mind that Billy had not contracted the disease. "I didn't feel justified in using the [antitoxin]," Welch would write a few weeks later in his medical report. "I had no idea what effect it might have." He and his nurse also decided to keep their tentative diagnosis to themselves, fearing it might send the community into a panic.

Instead, Welch rummaged through his pharmacy and pulled out all the old-fashioned remedies doctors had used to treat diphtheria before the invention of antitoxin in 1891. In a series of treatments, he gave Billy stimulants to strengthen his heart against the possible onslaught of toxin, which circulated in the bloodstream and attacked vital organs. He swabbed the child's throat with chloride of iron, an astringent that effectively broke up the lesions. These were not sure-fire cures, but in conjunction with the body's own immune system, they might provide a fighting chance.

The treatment seemed to work for a while: just hours after Welch swabbed the child's throat, the lesions had sloughed off and the color had returned to his cheeks. He was sleeping more comfortably and

---

1. There is some debate over Welch's notion about the inefficacy and the instability of the antitoxin. His fears that administering the antitoxin would weaken the boy were probably unfounded.

appeared stronger by the hour, and Welch recalled that the child's general condition became almost normal.

Then, by around 4:00 P.M. on Tuesday, Billy had taken a turn for the worse. Looking in on his young patient, the doctor faced his worst fears. It was diphtheria, clear and simple. The child was the very picture of the advanced stages of the disease: sunken eyes, an expression of unrelenting despair, dark lips the color of wild berries, like the ones the children brought in from the tundra. Each time Billy Barnett tried to draw air into his lungs, he coughed up blood.

At 6:00 P.M., the nurses called Welch back to the boy's bedside, and he saw that Billy was turning blue from a lack of oxygen and laboring ever harder for breath. He was in a state of collapse. Without using the antitoxin, there was nothing Welch could do. By now, it was even questionable whether an injection of fresh serum could save the child, given the late diagnosis and advanced stage of the disease. Welch had no alternative but to stand by and watch the boy shut down. Billy stared back up at him in fear. As the end approached, the child's windpipe clogged up and they could hear a faint, high-pitched trill, as if someone was slowly letting the air out of a balloon.

It was over. Welch made arrangements for the body's disposal, and went home. There was little else he could do that night, but in the morning he would have to make a full report to the town fathers. The coffin to hold the 40-pound body was a little over three feet long.

The short walk home down Front Street from the hospital on C Street and Second Avenue was tiring and cold: it was late and 14 degrees below, and most of Nome was already home, sitting close to the stove with a winter cache of books and old newspapers, or a stack of cards. The clapboards rattled and you could hear the ice popping out at sea, and on the street there was the sound of Eli Nicholi's horse as the man made his nightly rounds emptying the outhouse honey buckets.

Welch was not the first doctor to be caught off guard by diphtheria. Its onset was similar to other ailments of the throat, particularly tonsillitis, and its symptoms were varied, depending upon the severity of the outbreak and the health of the child. An outbreak in any community would have been a heavy weight for any small-town doctor, even one with sufficient antitoxin at hand; denial would not have been an unusual reaction. "In several cases I had to change the diagnosis and use the antitoxin after I *had tried to make myself believe* it was 'tonsillitis,' " wrote one Iowa doctor in 1896. For many, the diagnosis was simply too horrifying to accept.

In 1925, most doctors relied on visual aids to diagnose diphtheria. If there was any doubt, they then performed a throat culture, which could positively identify the rod-shaped diphtheria bacilli and determine the presence of toxin. Welch had little, if any, firsthand experience visually diagnosing diphtheria and even less making throat cultures. While Maynard Columbus may have been the best-equipped hospital in the region, its technology was of the most basic sort and its resources were limited at best. Electricity was unreliable and there was neither a laboratory nor an incubator for cultures. It had been years since Welch had done this type of work, and as he himself would admit, "I hardly feel competent."

THROUGH HIS medical journals, Welch had access to information about the symptoms of diphtheria and its various outbreaks across the United States. Despite the development of antitoxin, epidemics of diphtheria continued to occur in the 1920s, although at a much slower pace, infecting about 150,000 people annually and claiming 15,000 lives.

Before antitoxin, the death toll from diphtheria was dramatically higher, and it was one of the major causes of death in the United States as well as a leading killer of young children. The disease had wiped out communities in Europe and the Middle East; in 1735, an outbreak of a "plague in the throat" occurred in the American colonies, and continued for five fatal years. One historian estimated that 2,500 people out of every 100,000 died from the epidemic, a death toll that led to fears that the disease would destroy the colonies. Some towns lost nearly half of all their children.

The pious colonists struggled to explain how and why they were being stricken by diphtheria. The disease appeared to strike at random. No one understood that it could be spread by a healthy carrier, and when no amount of vigil, prayer, or good behavior could the save the children, at least one minister concluded that the mysterious plague was one of "the woeful effects of Original Sin."

Jonathan Dickinson of Massachusetts, an influential religious leader in the colonies, described the struggles his patients underwent:

> It frequently begins with a slight Indisposition, much resembling an ordinary Cold with a listless Habit, a slow and scarce discernable Fever, some soreness of the Throat and Tumefaction of the Tonsils: and perhaps a running of the Nose, the Countenance pale, and the eyes dull and heavy. The patient is not confined, nor any Danger apprehended for Days, till the Fever gradually increases, the whole Throat, and sometimes the Roof of the Mouth and Nostrils are covered with cankerous Crust. . . . When the lungs are thus affected, the Patient is first afflicted with a dry hollow Cough, which quickly succeeded with an extraordinary distressing asthmatic Symptoms and difficulty of Breathing, under which the poor miserable creature struggles, until released by a perfect Suffocation, or Stoppage of the Breath.

For the few who survived under Dickinson's care, the road to recovery was frightening and often left them with severe secondary infections and complications. "All that I have seen get over this dreadful Symptom . . . ," the minister wrote, "have by their perpetual Cough expectorated incredible Quantities of a tough whitish slough from their Lungs, for a considerable Time together. And on the other Hand, I have seen large Pieces of Crust, several inches Long and near an Inch broad, torn from the Lungs by the vehemence of the Cough. . . ."

Over the course of the next two decades, diphtheria continued to strike fear into the hearts of parents and physicians. The disease became endemic in many cities, and outbreaks were common. Physicians and researchers focused their attention on diphtheria, but no matter how well they understood its whims and manifestations, there was no cure. In sickbeds and in doctors' offices across the country, a child with a common sore throat could become an object of fear and panic.

Doctors tried every available salve, but most of these served only to prolong the patient's suffering or to hasten his or her death. Some physicians injected mercury, others swabbed or injected carbolic acid into the membrane or tried to forcibly remove the membrane with forceps, leaving behind a raw and bleeding surface upon which the bacteria fed. The more desperate resorted to sucking out the alien membrane to clear the airway of a suffocating child.

In the early 1820s, doctors began trying out a new procedure called tracheotomy, cutting through the muscles of the neck and into the airway. This was often as fatal as the disease, and the practice was discontinued in the 1880s after a New York doctor, Joseph O'Dwyer, developed small hollow tubes that could be inserted through the mouth into the windpipe. The O'Dwyer tube reduced the mortality of laryngeal diphtheria, a severe form of diphtheria, from virtually 100 percent to 75 percent.

A 75 percent mortality rate, however, was small comfort. The tubes were difficult to use. In addition, a child who could now breathe with the use of the tube could still suffer from the shutdown of the renal, respiratory, and eventually pulmonary systems caused by circulating toxin. As doctors labored, mothers who had watched the suffering of their loved ones sent letters to Louis Pasteur at his institute in Paris, urging him to find a cure. "You have done all the good a man could do on earth," one mother wrote. "If you will, you can surely find a remedy for the horrible disease called diphtheria. Our children to whom we teach your name as that of a great benefactor, will owe their lives to you."

Finally, a Prussian army surgeon named Emil Behring, building upon the work of the Pasteur Institute, developed an "anti-toxic" that could neutralize the diphtheria toxin. It was first used on a child in 1891, and it saved the child's life.

WELCH KNEW the odds were stacked against him if he did not find a fresh supply of serum. The disease was highly contagious. The bacteria were resilient and could survive for weeks on a piece of candy, a countertop, or a mitten. With a single touch, the bacteria could move from one warm body to the next; a single sneeze or a cough could carry the disease through the air; and a simple inhalation could mean death. In every corner of Nome, bacteria could be lying in wait for the touch of a child; every windowsill or schoolbook was a potential landing zone.

Welch also realized that the disease could move quickly beyond the town's boundaries and on to other coastal villages. As acting assistant surgeon of the U.S. Public Health Service and the territory's assistant commissioner of health, he was responsible for the welfare of some ten thousand people in Northwest Alaska, with jurisdiction reaching as far north as the Arctic coast and as far south as the Yukon River delta.

Most northwestern Alaskans were Eskimo, and they were at greatest risk. They had little natural resistance to any of the bacterial or viral illnesses brought in by seafarers or miners, and over the past one and a half centuries—since the first contact with Eurpeans—an astonishingly large portion of the population had succumbed to measles, tuberculosis, and flu.

Welch had witnessed the flu pandemic of 1918–19, which obliterated entire villages and settlements throughout Seward Peninsula. "The Natives showed absolutely no resistance," said the then Alaskan governor, Thomas Riggs. By the time the scourge was over, 8 percent of the total Native population in Alaska and 50 percent of the Native population in Nome had died. Those who survived continued to suffer from weakened immune systems.

During other epidemics of smallpox, measles, and typhoid fever, Welch's predecessors had set up quarantines and pesthouses to monitor and care for sick Natives. Native Alaskans had a well-grounded and paralyzing fear of disease. Eskimos believed in the spirit of death and feared that if a person died in their home that spirit would claim them next. A death often caused family members to panic and flee, and this only served to spread the disease.

Welch worried that Nome's Native population would react in the same way and that, in their attempts to flee, they would spread the bacteria through the town and down the coast.

. . .

THE NEXT MORNING, on Wednesday, January 21, Welch was shaken from his troubled sleep well before dawn. The daughter of Henry Stanley, an Eskimo on the Sandspit, was very sick and needed immediate attention. The family lived a mile and a half away; Welch decided it might be faster to walk than to hitch up the dogs and drive there. Gathering up his medical kit and his squirrel-skin parka and white cotton anorak with the red trim, he ran down the stairs and out onto the street.

The Sandspit was a long, thin strip of beach that ended at the mouth of the Snake River on the west side of town. Most Natives lived in single-room sod houses made of driftwood, whalebone, sod, scraps of tin, and whatever else they could salvage from the beach. Some of the homes were still lit by seal-oil lamps and the air inside was thick with the smell of seal, dried salmon, sweat, and damp fur. Welch was used to the smell and he had learned, over the years, to accept and even to admire the "strong, elemental" nature of these Natives. "They know how to be loyal, how to love, if not how to use table knives," he had written.

Seven-year-old Bessie Stanley lay in the back of the igloo, dark eyes peering out from a hollow-cheeked face, her chest heaving beneath an invisible weight. Welch took her temperature and found that the girl was feverish. Beads of sweat had broken out on her butter-colored skin, cutting rivulets through the grime.

Welch hovered over the girl, and as soon as he pried open her mouth, he could smell the stench. The inside of Bessie's mouth had become "one mass of fetid, stinking membrane," and when he touched the membrane, it bled profusely.

By late evening, the girl would be dead, and there was little doubt in Welch's mind that they were face to face with a catastrophic epidemic: the town was hovering on the edge of the abyss.[2]

2. Reports in the *Nome Nugget* at the time erroneously refer to this child as Richard Stanley. Medical records, however, show that a little girl named Bessie Stanley passed away.

He reached the apartment just as Lula was preparing lunch, and he sat down and covered his face with his hands. It took him a moment or two to gather up his thoughts and regain his professional composure. He told Lula what was happening, then picked up the phone and asked the operator to get the mayor, George Maynard, on the line as quickly as she could. Then he told Maynard to gather up the town council, every one of them, and immediately head on up to the hospital. There was no time to lose.

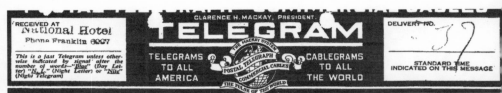

CLARENCE H. MACKAY, PRESIDENT.

TELEGRAM

TELEGRAMS
TO ALL
AMERICA

CABLEGRAMS
TO ALL
THE WORLD

DELIVERY NO.

STANDARD TIME
INDICATED ON THIS MESSAGE

NOME ALASKA JANUARY 22, 1925

CUMMING PUBHEALTH WASH DC

AN EPIDEMIC OF DIPHTHERIA IS ALMOST INEVITABLE HERE STOP I AM IN URGENT
NEED OF ONE MILLION UNITS OF DIPHTHERIA ANTOTOXIN STOP MAIL IS ONLY FORM OF
TRANSPORTATION STOP I HAVE MADE APPLICATION TO COMMISSIONER OF HEALTH OF
THE TERRITORIES FOR ANTITOXIN ALREADY STOP THERE ARE ABOUT 3000 WHITE
NATIVES IN THE DISTRICT

WELSH RELIEF STATION 295

M
H DIV.
Domestic Quar.

The telegram telling the world that icebound Nome had been stricken with diphtheria.
(U.S. Public Health Records, National Archives RG 90)

3

Quarantine

"Their [Alaskan Natives'] country is being over-run by strangers, the game slaughtered and driven away, the streams depleted of fish; hitherto unknown and fatal diseases brought to them, all which combine to produce a state . . . which must result in their extinction. Action in their interest is demanded by every consideration of justice and humanity."

—PRESIDENT THEODORE ROOSEVELT,
MESSAGE TO CONGRESS, DECEMBER 7, 1904.

I T WAS a comfortable office by Nome's standards, with a big bay window, a row of potted plants tenderly cared for by Head Nurse Emily Morgan, and shelves filled with the well-thumbed volumes of Welch's medical library. The room faced south onto the street and had a clear view of traffic. Welch often sat there and watched the whole town go by.

He knew every member of the town council. He had treated each of them, and their families as well, and on several occasions he and Lula had been invited to their homes for dinner. Most of them had children and none of them realized what was about to happen.

George Maynard was there, the burly publisher of the *Nome Nugget* and the town's mayor, and so was Mark Summers, superintendent of the Hammon Consolidated Gold Fields. The attorney Hugh O'Neil was also present, along with G. J. Lomen, the former mayor of Nome and now a judge, whose family was one of the most prominent in town.

Summers, thoughtfully, had shut down operations over at the Hammon mining camps so that his employees could take the day off to mourn young Billy's death and pay their respects to the child's father, who was a company employee.

Welch took a deep breath and began to explain what had taken place over the past few months, beginning with the numerous cases of sore throat he had begun to notice after the *Alameda* had sailed off and navigation shut down, moving to the young Eskimo child from Holy Cross, then on to the death of Margaret Eide. He had come to the conclusion that all of Nome's children were at risk. Billy Barnett had died of diphtheria, and there was every indication that out on the Sandpit the Eskimo girl, Bessie Stanley, was suffering from the same illness and would soon face the same fate. Welch could not say how any of them had contracted the disease, but it was clear to him that Nome now had an epidemic on its hands.

Futhermore, Welch fully expected that, given the contagious nature of the disease, new cases would begin to appear within twenty-four hours. The only treatment available for diphtheria was serum, he told them, and he had only enough for about six patients, at best. To make matters worse, those estimated 80,000 units were already six years old. Welch had ordered a fresh supply over the summer, but the units had failed to arrive on board the *Alameda*, and he could not expect another delivery until spring.

That morning, despite his earlier misgivings about the effects of the aged serum, he had injected Bessie Stanley with 6,000 units. He doubted this would have much effect because the girl had been treated too late after the symptoms had first appeared. In that regard, he was right: Bessie died several hours later.

To properly fight the epidemic, Welch said, he needed at least 1 million units.

Welch did not need to argue his case. It had been seven years earlier, in the fall of 1918, when the influenza virus was carried aboard the *Victoria* and brought ashore amidst the confusion of crates and supplies.

Time had literally stopped during the epidemic: the man responsible for winding the Segerstrom & Heger clock in front of the jewelry store had either died or left on the last boat, and no one bothered to reset it. The judge, the fire chief, the U.S. Marshal—even the town doctor who preceded Welch—had all beome infected and soon became too sick to work. (The other doctor fled aboard the *Victoria*.) Those who remained healthy were paralyzed with apprehension.

"It was impossible to get anyone to help those who were sick," wrote one survivor. "Those who were not sick were scared to death and would do nothing."

Nome's deputy marshal took charge of relief efforts, gathering up volunteers and sending them out to hunt for survivors. They had broken down doors and taken out the sickest of them, and brought in drums filled with stew to the Sandspit to feed the Eskimos. They had crashed through narrow openings into the darkened sod igloos and found entire families dead, some still sitting up in their chairs frozen in place after the fire had gone out. Others lay naked on the floor.

There was speculation that many of them had burned up with fever and stripped off their clothes to cool down. Children, some barely alive, lay between their dead parents for warmth. In one eight-day period, 162 Natives had died on the Sandspit, and a once bustling and lively community fell silent. The smoke no longer wafted up from the stovepipes, and there was no one left with strength enough to stoke the fires that had kept the igloos warm.

"Natives dying every few minutes," said one urgent dispatch from Nome to Alaskan officials.

Rescuers had to fight off starving dogs to reach the living as well as the dead. With no one left to feed them, the animals had turned on their masters. One Eskimo was found dead in the center of his dwelling with his hands frozen to his rifle, pointed toward the door. He had frozen to death trying to fend off the dogs.

In just a few weeks, the virus spread to the communities along Northwest Alaska. Relief parties moved by dogsled from village to deserted village in a desperate search for those still alive. Rescuers managed to save a girl and her infant sister, who had been trapped inside their igloo for days while starving dogs, teeth bared, paced outside. The girl had survived huddled next to her dead mother. She would occasionally put her arm out of the entrance of the igloo and scrape up a little snow, which she would warm in her mouth and then give to her sister. Another Native child was found with his feet frozen to the floor. He had sacrificed his mukluks to his younger sister.

A mission house at Pilgrim Hot Springs about fifty miles north of Nome took on the aspect of a wartime triage unit. "Were it within your power to pay me a visit," the Pilgrim missionary wrote, "you would find my house filled with orphans and sick people. Near by, in a tent, you would see seven corpses. At six miles from here, scattered in different igloos, you would see 40 other corpses. You are horrified? Hardly was the ordeal over in Nome, when I learned that my flock up here had the disease. I hurried up to help. Twenty-three were already dead. I gathered 30 in my house. Seven died on my hands. The others are convalescent. I am alone with a good man, but one old and feeble. I do not know how to take care of babies and small children. What else can we do?"

The sickness left terrible emotional scars on Nome's survivors, many of whom were housed in an old schoolhouse on Steadman and Third Avenue. There, in a gymnasium that had been turned into an aid station, two Natives committed suicide. The first hung himself from a coatrack while his friend watched and then the other took the noose and put it around his own neck. The *Nome Nugget* reported that the second body was found swinging in front of a blackboard on which the Natives had written a suicide note in chalk: they wished only to end their lives quickly.

When the virus had finally run its course, volunteers began burying the dead. Bodies were removed by dogsled and piled up in abandoned houses until the spring, when a mass grave could be dug in the thawed ground. Cabins, furs, bedding, and clothes were burned as a protective measure. Dogs were shot, and for the first time in Nome's recorded history, the evening malamute chorus was silent.

The flu had taken the lives of at least one thousand people in the Nome vicinity and more than two thousand in all of Alaska. Of the three hundred children orphaned in the territory, ninety were in Nome—the large majority of them Eskimo.

The Natives were "mowed down like grass," said one missionary.

Everyone at the council meeting remembered the epidemic, and each had vivid memories of the devastation. Mayor Maynard immediately asked Welch to take charge of the situation. Instead, Welch suggested that a temporary Board of Health with the power to act independently of the town council be established. The council approved, and Maynard, Welch, and Hammon superintendent Mark Summers became the principal members of the board. Without further prompting from Welch, they all agreed on a single course of action: to lock down the town straight away. Welch suggested that every school, church, moviehouse, and lodge be shut down, and that travel along the trails be strongly discouraged and banned outright for children.

One council member remembered that a card party was in full swing over at Pioneer Hall, and they agreed that someone should go over and shut it down. Then, in an effort to break the news gently to his fellow citizens and keep panic down to a minimum, Mayor Maynard decided to print up a circular detailing the facts of the epidemic as well as the first suggested steps to a total quarantine.

The meeting was over. The town leaders stood up and the health board made plans to meet again every evening until the danger had passed. It was late afternoon by the time Welch headed out. He made his way to the radio telegraph station and asked the U.S. Signal Corps officer in charge to send out two urgent bulletins: one was to be coded for all points in Alaska and would alert every major town and official, including the governor in Juneau, to Nome's desperate need for serum.

The other would go to Washington, D.C., to Welch's colleagues at the U.S. Public Health Service, which regulated the production of antitoxins and vaccines:

An epidemic of diphtheria is almost inevitable STOP I am in urgent need of one million units of diphtheria antitoxin STOP Mail is only form of transportation STOP I have made application to Commissioner of Health of the Territories for antitoxin already STOP

In less than a week, Nome's plight would make the front pages of nearly every newspaper in America.

THE QUARANTINE began almost immediately. The Dream Theatre was closed and all social gatherings disrupted. Welch told his good friends the Walshes to pack up their belongings and head out to their isolated cabin a few miles beyond Nome and ordered them not to return until they'd heard from him.

Schoolchildren were ordered to go home, and Jean Summers-Wolf remembered much later that she and the other children knew right away that something was radically wrong. "I remember holding my breath real tight and running past any building I encountered with that big red sign QUARANTINE. KEEP OUT."

Maynard finished composing his notice and sent it out to be posted all over town, then headed for his office at the *Nome Nugget* to make sure it made the next edition. He had written it carefully, but the soothing tone had failed to mask entirely the darker implications.

> An epidemic of diphtheria has broken out in Nome and if proper precautions are taken there is no cause for alarm. On the other hand, if parents do not keep their children isolated from other children, the epidemic may spread to serious proportions. . . . All children should be compelled to wash their faces and hands frequently during the day with some mild soap such as Ivory Soap. A strong soap is worse than none at all as it has a tendency to cause the face and hands to chap and crack and render them easily susceptible to the diphtheria germ . . . every effort will be made on the part of officials to prevent the carriers of the disease from leaving Nome and thereby contaminating the adjacent camps.

Despite their attempts to contain the disease, the health board had acted too late. Soon after Bessie's Stanley's death, her sisters, Dora and Mary, had developed membranes in their throats and their parents also appeared to have developed related symptoms. Welch treated them all "vigorously with the old serum."

By Saturday, January 24, the fourth day of the crisis, the death toll stood at four, by conservative estimates, and still there was no word of any available serum from Fairbanks, Anchorage, or Juneau, Alaska's major towns, or from Washington, D.C.

The phone in Welch's office began to ring with one parent after another calling in about a sick child or a loved one: Lars Rynning, the young superintendent of schools, called to say he had a sore throat and a fever of 99.6, and that he was particularly worried about an ulceration that had begun to form in his throat. His wife also complained of a bad sore throat, and both were worried about the effect all this might have on their two-month-old son.

Welch came over and examined the infant and told the Rynnings that, as near as he could tell, their son was in good health. Mother's milk contains a natural immunity to diphtheria and very young infants stand a 90 percent chance of fighting off the disease without medication. Welch was convinced that the Rynnings had been exposed to the virus and in an effort to protect their son, he placed the parents under quarantine. But he decided against giving them any of the precious serum. They were young and strong and he felt they stood a better chance of survival than most others. The medicine had to be saved for the worst cases, and there would be many more.

There was one other detail about Lars Rynning which bothered Welch: Rynning was not only the school superintendent but a teacher as well, and the chances were high that he had already come into contact with nearly every school-age child in Nome.

Welch was already feeling overwhelmed and exhausted, and there was no one around to replace him. The nearest doctor was four hundred miles away, a ten-day journey by dogsled. "My nurses are the only consultants I have," he noted in his medical report.

EMILY MORGAN was without doubt the most efficient and outstanding nurse in Welch's employ, and she had already proven her worth. She had had a long career in public nursing. For three years she had served with the Red Cross in a mobile hospital on the western front in France, working amid the chaos of bombs and the arrival of the dying and wounded. When the war ended she returned home to Wichita, Kansas, to continue her practice.

Morgan was forty-seven when she arrived in Nome the previous fall from Unalaska, on the Aleutian Chain, where she had provided medical care to the Native community. She was nearly a foot taller than Welch and provided a cheerful, easygoing counterpoint to her boss. She also had firsthand experience with diphtheria: she had been infected back in Wichita and spent three weeks in bed, and by the time she'd recovered from it she knew every twist and turn of its terrible progression.

It was time for Morgan to go to work. At Welch's suggestion, the health board had appointed her Quarantine Nurse, and she would go out in her heavy woolen sweater, fur parka, and knee-high fur boots to find and treat the most severe cases. She soon found herself putting up more and more of the red and black QUARANTINE signs, which hung over the doorways and stood out against the white of the snow.

Morgan focused on the Sandspit, where teams of teachers and volunteers handed out food, fuel, and water. She had learned to work in the crudest and most insalubrious environments and thought nothing of roughing it out in the cold. But Nome was particularly tough. In Kansas, she said, "we had plenty of doctors and hospitals," but here she often worked alone, with Welch only occasionally at her side.

Morgan always brought along her medical bag, which contained a clinical thermometer, tongue depressors, several tubes of antitoxin, some candy to tempt the children, and a flashlight. She checked in constantly on her patients and took care to see that the antitoxin was working, but often found she could offer only her sympathy.

Once, on her rounds, Morgan returned to the home of an Eskimo family and was disturbed by the condition of one of the five children, a young girl named Mary, whose symptoms were extreme: the child's tonsils were covered with a membrane, the darkest Morgan had ever seen. As Morgan approached the igloo, a young Eskimo boy came running out.

"You are too late," he told her. "Mary has gone to heaven."

Inside, Morgan found the father hewing a coffin out of rough boards while his two other daughters looked on. Morgan could do little to ease their grief, so she knelt beside the father and "did all I could toward finishing the crude box." When they were done, the man lined the box with his daughter's parka, placed her inside, nailed it shut, and buried her in a nearby snowdrift. A proper burial would have to wait until spring, when the ground had thawed out.

Morgan visited one family after another. During one house call to a young girl named Vivian Blackjack, Morgan noticed that while the parents sat cross-legged in the middle of the room eating dried fish dipped in seal oil, their daughter lay under the covers in her bunk.

"Her sharp black eyes stared at me defiantly; her lips were compressed tightly. I knew by the redness of her face that her temperature was high," she remembered. Morgan tried to open the girl's mouth but she resisted.

"I smiled at her and in a low tone told her mother I would not force her. But with a temperature of 104 something had to be done . . . then in a pleading voice [Vivian] said, 'Mother, let us pray.' "

Kneeling by the bedside, Morgan prayed with the mother and child, and when Vivian "looked straight at me and opened her mouth . . . her throat showed all the indications of diphtheria."

Morgan gave the child a shot of serum, and her condition improved. But both Morgan and Welch estimated that at the current rate of infection, their stock of serum would not last through the week. Without a new supply, many would die.

Late on Saturday evening, Morgan and Welch went to the health board to summarize their findings. Between them, they said, they had about twenty confirmed cases, with at least fifty others still at risk.

The board had been briefed on Welch's desperate message to Washington, and while all knew there was nothing more they could do to help the government find serum, there was another problem they might solve—how to get serum to Nome once it was located. The Bering Sea was icebound so a sea trip direct from Seattle was out of the question. That left the land route. At this time of year mail and supplies were shipped by boat to the ice-free port of Seward in southeast Alaska, then traveled north for 420 miles to Nenana on the only major railroad in Alaska. From there it took about twenty-five days for the mail teams to travel the 674 miles west to Nome. It was a start-and-stop route, divided up among several drivers, with time built in for overnight rests. The board had to come up with a faster alternative.

Mark Summers had a plan, an express delivery. The entire route could be covered by two fast dogsled teams, one starting from the railhead at Nenana heading west, the other from Nome heading east. They would meet halfway on the trail at Nulato. Summers knew the one man who could do the western portion of the run, from Nome to Nulato and then back again: a scrappy Norwegian outdoorsman named Leonhard Seppala. Seppala was the gold company's main dog driver. He supervised the company's 110 miles of ditches that supplied water to the gold fields, and he freighted supplies and passengers out to the company's mining camps and ferried officials on business trips to other towns in Alaska. Tireless and disciplined in his work, he was undoubtedly the fastest musher in Alaska.

Seppala's record on the trail was legendary, earning him the nickname "King of the Trail." He had won most dog races he entered in Nome and in the Interior, and with his favorite lead dog, a well-known dog who went by the name of Togo, Seppala had toppled a number of long-distance records. Seppala knew every turn of the trail from Nome to Nenana and had once reached Fairbanks—the Interior capital seventy miles northeast of Nenana—in thirteen and a half days with the added weight of a passenger. It had taken him just four days to reach Nulato, halfway on the Nenana-to-Nome trail, and he had averaged an exhausting eighty-one miles per day.

After listening carefully to Summers's suggestion, the health board's approval was unanimous. But Maynard suggested that the board members also consider one other option: to fly in the serum.

The mayor had long been an advocate of Alaskan aviation. It was a fledgling industry in the territory, but he was certain that planes would eventually end the crippling isolation of many Alaskan towns and allow them to thrive.

While flying the serum in would be quicker, board members were openly skeptical: winter flights were extremely dangerous, the cockpits were wide open, and it would be a tough trip in the cold and the wind.

The previous year, a former army pilot had been the first to fly through the Alaskan winter. The experimental flights, which were air-mail runs between Fairbanks and McGrath, were considered a great success in Alaska and proved that winter flight in the territory was possible. But compared to the projected flight to Nome, the air-mail run had been relatively short and had taken place in much warmer weather.

That very evening Summers paid his employee a visit to tell him to prepare for the run of his life, and to let him know that although the board was considering an air rescue, most of them believed that Nome's fate lay in Seppala's hands. Meanwhile, Maynard sent a telegram to the one man who had the power and political clout to make an air rescue possible, Alaska's delegate to the U.S. Congress, Dan Sutherland. Sutherland had been working to bring aviation to Alaska for the past three years and had lobbied hard for the experimental air-mail runs.

> Serious epidemic of diphtheria has broken out here STOP No fresh antitoxin here STOP Interview surgeon general department of public health and tell him to dispatch million units antitoxin to Nome immediately. . . . Airplane would save time if feasible.

Now, as the delegate sat in his office near Capitol Hill and read the message from Nome's mayor, he saw a perfect opportunity to herald the cause of aviation once again.

It was time to send the birds up into the Alaskan sky.

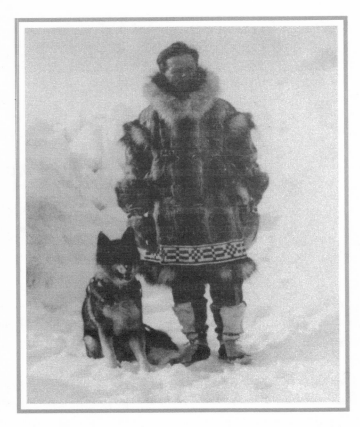

Veterans of the Trail: Leonhard Seppala and his trusted lead dog Togo.
(Carrie M. McLain Memorial Museum, Nome, Alaska)

4

Gone to the Dogs

"Any man can make friends with any dog but it takes a long time and mutual trust and mutual forbearance and mutual appreciation to make a partnership. Not every dog is fit to be partner with a man; nor every man, I think, fit to be partner with a dog."
— ARCHDEACON HUDSON STUCK

LEONHARD SEPPALA was forty-seven and by rights he should have been slowing down. But he was as strong as the day he arrived in Nome to search for gold in the summer of 1900, and even after a quarter century living and working in the cold, he was as agile and graceful as a gymnast. At five foot four and about 145 pounds, the King of the Trail didn't quite look the part. He had a rugged, youthful face and light brown hair thick with boyish waves that rode back over his head, as if perpetually blown by Nome's northern winds.

He was a rare natural athlete, a man of unusual strength and endurance who would have had no trouble keeping up with most professional sportsmen. While the majority of the dogsled drivers would have considered thirty miles to be a hard day's drive, Seppala often traveled fifty, sometimes even one hundred miles, weather permitting, logging twelve hours on the trail with a full load. One winter alone he covered 7,000 miles by dogsled.

In the summer, when most of the dogs were idle, Seppala would hitch his team up to a wheeled cart he called the "Pupmobile" and head out to the gold fields to do his job. He drove along an abandoned railway track and checked on a vast system of ditches that supplied water to thaw the ground ahead of the dredges. All year round, he stayed close to the animals.

His friends called him "Sepp," a peppy moniker for the cheerful Norwegian immigrant. He was something of a show-off, known to flip double back handsprings just for laughs and land with a somersault. He would walk down Front Street on his hands, his back arched and his mukluk Eskimo boots almost brushing his tousled head, and the schoolchildren would laugh and clap their hands.

Over the years, the only visible change was the number of wrinkles on his face, burnt into the skin by the cold, the trail winds, and the sun. When he smiled, which was often, the lines deepened and furrowed beneath the cheekbones and around the mouth, and radiated out from the eyes.

There had been relatively little snow this year, and so the dogs were not in their usual prime condition. Ever since Mark Summers's call for help, Seppala had been training with the team in the treeless hills that stretched away to the Sawtooth Mountains. The plan was for Seppala to travel more than three hundred miles to Nulato, almost midway between Nome and Nenana. It would be a long haul. So much was at stake, he thought, that at first he hesitated. This was not in character for the usually confident Seppala.

He had decided to train with twenty of the thirty-six Siberian Huskies in the kennel. This was a relatively large string for such a light load, but the dogs could turn sore-footed on the hard run to Nulato and some might even tire out. Seppala planned to drop several off at the villages along the trail, so that he could have fresh replacements for the return.

The trail between Nulato and Nome was one of Alaska's most hazardous. Much of it ran along the windswept, blizzard-prone coast of Norton Sound, and the most dangerous stretch was a forty-two-mile shortcut across the sound. Depending on the conditions under which the sound froze, the shortcut could be either a long stretch of glare ice—a slippery sheen that had been ground down by wind and blowing sand—or a course littered with giant pieces of ice rubble, crevices, and long avenues of tiny spears of ice that could shred a dog's paws into bloody ribbons.

The biggest risk in taking the shortcut, however, was getting separated from shore: with little warning, the ice could break up and carry a team away into the Bering Sea in silent, counterclockwise circles.

On and off the trail, the dogs required constant attention, and Seppala poured time and money into his huskies. He had raised each of them from the time they were pups and he knew them as well as he knew his wife and child. He fed and cared for them and sometimes ate with them, tearing off hunks of dried salmon with his teeth.

"The dogs always came first in importance," Constance, his wife of fifty-two years, told a newspaper reporter in 1954. ". . . Our living room was often a place of utter confusion, littered with mukluks, harnesses, dog sleds, tow lines, ropes and other equipment being repaired and spliced and generally worked over."

Food was a constant concern for the drivers of Alaska. The dogs' diet had to include enough protein and fat to keep them healthy and warm for winter travel, and the drivers needed to stock huge quantities. The most common food source was salmon. A musher would build fish traps out of wood and wire and lay them out in the river to catch the salmon runs.[1] Then he would cut up the fish and hang them out to dry on racks. The job could take a whole summer; each year the driver would stock about 5,000 pounds of the vitamin-rich meat.

The dogs' health and attitude had to be monitored on a daily basis, whether the animals ran or not; an unchecked virus could easily spread and wipe out an entire kennel. On the trail, every dog's paws had to be checked and, when necessary, treated, and the relative strength of each animal taken into account. One dog's special trait

---

1. Many of the drivers used a fish wheel, which had two baskets attached to a long wooden axle. As the wheel turned in the current of the river, migrating fish were scooped up by the baskets and dropped down a ramp that led into a compartment. The fish wheel was held in place by an anchor on shore or by posts driven into the riverbed.

could be a boon on a particular section of the trail but a hazard on another. A good driver had to put his dogs' needs ahead of his own.

Mushing was the easiest part of the job. After a ten-hour day on the trail, the animals were the first to eat, and preparations could take two or three hours. Wood had to be chopped and holes hacked through the ice for water, which was then hauled up to the camp pail by pail—a gallon for each dog. If there was no water, a driver had to go through the tedious process of melting snow in a pot; it took 4 quarts of snow to produce a single quart of water.

Along the coast, the driver would feed the dogs strips of dried salmon, bones included, and if there was enough wood around, he would cook up a thick fish soup (some drivers preferred beaver meat, which was also rich in fat) with rice or oatmeal. On the trail, each of Seppala's dogs was given a pound of dried salmon and a third of a pound of seal blubber a day.

Once the feeding was over, the animals' sore muscles were massaged and boughs of spruce were cut down for their bedding. The smell and feel of it was a comfort to the animals, whose well-being was an important factor on the long hauls. A tired and discouraged animal could turn a simple trail into an obstacle course. The dogs seemed to appreciate every act of kindness, and they relaxed and settled down after their meal. This was followed by a ritual the mushers referred to as "the thank-you howl."

It began with a single dog's high-pitched, dreamlike wail, which was picked up by a second and then a third dog. Soon, every dog had its nose up, joining in a full-throated cacophony. The singing would end as suddenly as it began, and the dogs would begin to turn in ever-tightening circles, pawing at their bedding until they were comfortable. Then they would cover their noses with their tails and fall asleep. Finally the driver would have a few moments to take care of his own needs.

Seppala had loved the work from the moment he first stepped behind a sled in his early twenties, during his first winter in Nome. Jafet Lindeberg, one of the Three Lucky Swedes, had lured him to Alaska to work for his mining company, and had sent him out to look into rumors of a gold strike ninety miles northeast of town. Seppala had a clear recollection of that first run: he was mesmerized by the sway of the sled and the feel of runners gliding through the snow.

It took a good deal of strength to jerk the heavy sled around sharp curves and compensate for a slanted trail, and a fair amount of stamina to pedal the sled along flat ground and jog behind it, mile after mile, up sharp inclines and over rock and tundra.

It was wearing and often bone-crunching work, but occasionally it lent itself to reverie. A driver would be the only human being for miles, an extension of the landscape, and as he pedaled in rhythm to the dogs' gait, he became an extension of the team.

In the vast silence, Seppala could hear the patter of the dogs' feet on the crusted snow and their steady pant as they pulled ahead in the cold. There was something soothing about the sound of the sled in motion: the creak of the wood like the rigging of a schooner under full sail, the rub of the rawhide lashings, the swish of the runners on the snow. This was a broad terrain, an empty ocean, and when the weather behaved, the sled would glide easily over the trail's swells. The only marks left behind were two parallel lines in the snow and the clouds of the dogs' exhalations, which lingered over the trail for a moment.

"The birchwood runners of my sled make tracks so deep in my memory I can see them to this day," Seppala once said of his first dog team. "All [the dogs] asked at the end of a grueling day was to be fed."

The first rule of survival was to hang on to the team, because without the dogs you were dead.

SEPPALA TENSED up as he prepared for the trip to Nulato. He was apprehensive about the run, and the huskies could sense it. "Every time the telephone rang," Seppala said, "the dogs would hear it in the kennels and all tune up in an expectant howl. . . ."

Seppala was one of few Alaskan drivers who depended almost exclusively on Siberians. As far as Seppala was concerned, no other dog could equal the speed and stamina of his animals. He may have seen his reflection in the dogs: they were just as driven and competitive as he was, and they were smaller and lighter than their peers. The dogs could be playful and amusing; they could also be tough and unrelenting. A resident of Nome once found Seppala at work training his dogs, and remembered that one moment he was on the sled runners pedaling with his feet and throwing snowballs at them, and the next he was running beside them "like a reindeer." He and the dogs shared the same color eyes, the piercing, bluish-white of glacier ice. To be the object of Seppala's gaze could be an unsettling experience.

The present-day Siberian Husky came from east of the Lena River in Siberia, where Natives had used dog teams to hunt for fur-bearing animals, seal, and polar bear for centuries.[2] By the late seventeenth century, after the Russians had moved into the region to colonize it, dog driving in Siberia had become fairly sophisticated. The Natives were forced to pay taxes to the Russians, who often accepted dog-driving services in lieu of payment. Villagers were called on to transport officials to their fortified towns and outposts and carry goods to distant communities. Trading fairs also began to play an important role in the economic life of the region and many villagers had to travel distances of more than 1,000 miles with loaded sleds to barter for goods.

Traveling over mountain ranges, rivers, and tundra for a period of several decades, the dogs grew stronger and faster. Many of the Native groups practiced selective breeding: they would geld the inferior males, and only the elite—the fastest, strongest, and hardiest— were allowed to mate. By the late nineteenth century, the Siberian had become a tough cross-country dog, bred and built to cover long distances.

The Siberian dog was twice as fast and could travel at least twice as

2. Seppala—and many current Siberian owners—referred to the breed as "Siberians." "Husky" is a generic term for all double-coated, prick-eared breeds and was given to the Siberians when the American Kennel Club granted the dogs official recognition. According to Russ Tabbert's *Dictionary of Alaskan English*, the term Husky "developed in the 19th century from a shortened variant of 'Eskimo' used by English speakers as a name for Canadian Eskimos. Eskimo dogs were therefore known as 'Husky Dogs' which was shortened to 'Husky'" (p. 204).

far as its cousins on the other side of the Bering Strait. During a race between a merchant and a Russian officer in the Kolyma River region in 1869, one team covered 150 miles in fifteen hours; the other made it in sixteen hours. The malamute teams of Nome, which were bred for freighting heavy cargo, rarely went faster than five miles an hour.

The dogs of eastern Siberia caught the eye of the anthropologist Waldemar Bogoras, who traveled to the region around the turn of the century. Bogoras wrote about the Natives' training and disciplining of their dogs. Their training began as early as two months, and the puppies of a litter were often hitched up behind the mother to help them learn the commands. The teams of eastern Siberia had as many as fourteen dogs, hooked up in pairs on either side of the gang line. Bogoras noted that a strong and well-rested team could travel five hundred miles in ten days. After just two days' rest, they could get back on the trail with the same energy and survive on a daily ration of "a piece of blubber measuring two inches each way, and some shreds of putrid walrus meat or whale skin."

"The dogs," Bogoras said, "are quite unwearying."

When they were not working, the animals lived on even less. In the spring, when the maritime catch was less abundant, they were let loose to forage for scraps and to hunt, and this encouraged their feral nature. They hunted for mice and ground squirrel, and sniffed out and devoured dead salmon on the southern shores of the Bering. Only the strongest and those with the slowest metabolism survived.

The huskies, like many of the Native sled dogs of the north, such as the Malamute of Alaska and the Inuit dogs of Greenland, survived in the cold because of an extraordinary combination of physical features. They had two coats—an outer one made of long, coarse guard hairs that protected the skin against water, snow, and sun; and an undercoat of soft, dense, and wooly fur for warmth. The undercoat resembled the down found in parkas and was shed during the summer. The ability of northern sled dogs to retain heat is considerable: because dogs sweat through the pads of their feet, the chance of heat radiating through their skin and two thick coats is virtually nil. The tail is well furred and bushy, and curls over the dog's nose while he sleeps, providing protection from the cold. (The tail also protects the groin area, the one place on a husky where there is little, if any, fur.)

The eyes tend to be almond-shaped, so there is less exposure to the wind and snow, and the ears are pricked and covered with soft fur on the inside to minimize heat loss. The paws are slightly oval and the pads tough and compact to minimize the buildup of ice, which can lacerate and cripple a dog. These dogs can withstand temperatures of minus 80 degrees.

IT IS difficult to say when the first Siberian dog stepped onto soil in North America. Trade between Siberian and Alaskan Natives was not uncommon, and it is probable that some dogs were included in trades. But it is believed that the first time these dogs were brought across the Bering Strait to race in North America was in 1908. The race was the All Alaska Sweepstakes. A fur trader in Nome named William Goosak heard about dogs in the Anadyr delta who could travel at nine miles an hour for eleven straight hours. Goosak journeyed across the Bering Strait and brought a team back for the competition in 1909. In Nome, the dogs quickly became the butt of jokes. They were puny compared to the local malamutes—nearly half the size—and looked more like foxes than wolves. They were docile, even timid, and were laughingly referred to as "Siberian rats."[3] Once in harness, however, they made a different impression. Although small, they were almost always identical in size, and their smooth, unified gait seemed effortless. Nome's malamutes, by contrast, had a more varied background, and it was harder to find a team similar in size and reach. The malamutes could not pull as efficiently at their top speed.

Goosak felt confident that his Siberians could trounce the competition and he hired a driver to race them. Goosak, however, was alone

3. The Siberian Husky's relatively small size made it an efficient puller at fast speeds. Newfoundlands and Malamutes are too large to pull sleds quickly over long distances. Big dogs have proportionately less muscle and bone than small dogs and tire out more easily over long distances. In addition, they have more trouble getting rid of excess heat.

in his opinion. The odds weighed so heavily against him in 1909 that had he won the race, it would have broken the bank in Nome. His team fared poorly against the twelve other competitors, a failure due in large part to the driver's racing techniques. The driver was not a skilled strategist and failed to choose the right times to pace, rest, and feed the dogs. When the team crossed the finish line, a few spectators noticed that the "rats" looked as fresh as when they had begun. Some of them even trotted up to people they recognized in the crowd, tails held high in the air with excitement.

Among those who were impressed was a wealthy aristocrat from Scotland named Fox Maule Ramsay. As soon as navigation opened in June, Ramsay chartered a schooner, sailed across the Bering Strait, and returned with some sixty Siberian Huskies "howling from every porthole." The dogs were from Markova, a Native trading center on the Anadyr River in northeastern Siberia.

In April 1910, Ramsay entered three teams in the third annual All Alaska Sweepstakes. A popular Finnish driver named "Iron Man" Johnson headed one of the teams, and few believed he stood a chance against Scotty Allan, Nome's most famous driver. "Iron Man" proved them wrong. Johnson crossed the finish line well ahead of the seven other drivers, setting a record that still stands: 74 hours, 14 minutes, and 37 seconds. With more than one hundred miles to go before the finish line, the "Iron Man" had gone snow-blind and had to rely on his blue-eyed leader, Kolyma, to take him across Death Valley. At one point in the race he became so exhausted that he had to strap himself to his sled. When the Sweepstakes Queen placed the victory wreath around Johnson's neck, the burly musher struggled off the sled and burst into tears. Giving all credit to his dogs, he placed the wreath around Kolyma and cried: "I did not win the race. This leader won it."

Despite the huskies' performance in 1910, many remained skeptical of the breed. Allan's malamutes won in 1911 and 1912, beating out many of the Siberian Husky teams, but Seppala never lost faith in the dogs, whose small size and muscular compactness resembled his own.

"There seems to be almost no limit to his [the breed's] endurance and his willingness to give all he has got in the way of strength and speed when he is called upon in an emergency," Seppala once said. "There is no other type of dog that I know of that can stand the mile eating pace that he hits up once he gets going."

These dogs simply needed the right driver.

The following year, Seppala would luck into his first Siberian Husky team, and it was his friend and boss Jafet Lindeberg who provided the stroke of good fortune. In 1913, Lindeberg had bought a team of Siberians as a gift for the explorer Roald Amundsen, who had been planning an expedition to the North Pole. Lindeberg asked Seppala to train the dogs, and the driver gladly accepted. "I literally fell in love with them from the start, and I could hardly wait for sledding snow to start their training." A few weeks after the puppies arrived, Amundsen canceled the trip, and Lindeberg turned the dogs over to Seppala.

By 1913, Seppala had built a reputation as a capable dog driver for Lindeberg's Pioneer Mining Company. As he began training the new dogs, he attracted the attention of Scotty Allan, who encouraged him to enter the race in 1914. Seppala had followed the races since the very beginning, and every evening after work he would head down to the Board of Trade Saloon to root for his favorites. He had always admired Allan from afar and had watched how that driver handled his dogs.

But Seppala had been undecided for weeks about whether or not to compete. His team was young and had little experience in difficult conditions. The only veteran was the freight leader, Suggen, a tough dog that was half Siberian and half malamute. There was also the question of stamina: Seppala was not sure if he was ready to drive for four days with little sleep and under the pressure of competition. The wind, the cold, and the distance were so tough that one in three drivers gave up or arrived at the finish line hurt or "raving mad."

"It was truly a land where the Devil himself held sway," Seppala once said.

A sampling of dispatches from the racecourse coming in to the Board of Trade could send shivers down any aspirant's back. "Three miles this side of Solomon. Rope tied around waist dragging his team against the blizzard," said one, which described a competitor named

Coke Hill, who had given Allan a run for his money in 1911. Few drivers had time to eat. "Iron Man" Johnson claimed to have eaten just two hard boiled eggs during his whole four-day ordeal in 1910. To help the dogs along, the drivers would often run behind the sleds for long stretches of the 408-mile course; the journey up the slopes and over the ice hummocks with hardly a bite of food exhausted most of them, and many suffered from hallucinations.[4]

One All Alaska Sweepstakes competitor spoke of seeing a phantom team of black horses racing ahead of the dogs. He began to shout at them to move out of the way and continued to do so all the way to the finish line. In the 1910 race, after falling down a 200-foot vertical cliff, Allan imagined he saw a lantern bobbing ahead of the team, and the vision guided him to the finish line. The lantern stayed with him until he was three and a half miles from Nome. Then he blacked out. "They told me I came in with five dogs hitched, two in the sled, and three tied behind," Allan said. "One has to finish with all his dogs in harness, in the sled, or attached to the sled. I don't remember tying the three loose dogs."[5]

WITH JUST a few weeks left to go until the race, Seppala decided to enter, which was a rash and almost fatal move. Neither he nor Suggen knew the trail.

4. Although trail and weather conditions can vary so widely that no race can ever be the same, it is interesting that in 1983, when five-time Iditarod champion Rick Swenson raced the course in an anniversary challenge, he placed first but came in ten hours short of the all-time record set in 1910 by Johnson. Swenson's winning time was the sixth fastest in sweepstakes history (*Dogs of the North* [Anchorage: Alaska Geographic Society, 1987], 68).
5. Putting an injured dog on a sled was standard practice among dog freighters and it became a rule in the race. The sweepstakes forbade cruel treatment. If a driver was caught breaking the rule, he was disqualified. It was common sense among good drivers that a well-cared-for dog worked harder than one who had been abused or intimidated. However, there were drivers who abused their dogs out of ignorance or plain cruelty, and the sweepstakes helped to improve the general treatment, care, breeding, and training of sled dogs.

At the start of the 1914 race Seppala was up against a tough field of competitors, which included Scotty Allan, "Iron Man" Johnson, and another notable musher named Fred Ayer. He felt nervous and excited. The weather was calm, and for the first forty miles the race went smoothly. Then a blizzard kicked up. It could not have happened at a worse moment. Seppala was on the summit of Topkok Mountain, and the dogs, pushed forward by a strong tailwind, appeared to have lost the trail.

"By the time we were making it seemed to me that unless I hit the Topkok cabin, we would run a chance of falling over the cliffs which lined the shore," he later recalled. Suddenly, in a lull in the storm, the clouds parted. Seppala's worst fear was about to come true.

Stretched out 600 feet below him was the Bering Sea. The edge of the cliff was less than 20 feet away. Seppala jumped on the sled brake, but the metal claws only skidded on the hard snow. He grabbed a steel bar he kept in his sled for emergencies, jammed it into a hole in the brake board, then leaned on it with all his weight. The sled came to a stop. The dogs were now facing downward on an icy slope just feet away from the edge of the cliff. The puppies strained to keep going forward. Still leaning on the bar, Seppala shouted calmly to Suggen over the noise of the wind and ordered him to turn the team around. Suggen growled at the young dogs, but they were reluctant to swing the sled away from the cliff and into the wind. Seppala considered leaving them behind and climbing up the slope, but "the more I thought it over the less I could consider leaving my dogs to face such a tragic fate," he told a reporter later.

Seppala urged the lead dog to force the team around, and Suggen understood the task. He growled again and moved to make the turn. Timidly, then more confidently, the young dogs began to follow, one by one. Suggen leaned into his harnesses, belly close to the ground, as the team clawed its way up the slope. By now, the icy crust was tearing and ripping apart the dogs' paws.

"I don't know what [Suggen] told them but it worked. I have never been able to figure out whether dogs think or not, but every once in awhile some incident like this makes me wonder," Seppala said.

Seppala scratched from the race. He was ashamed of himself, but he had learned one or two things about sled dogs and sled racing. The trail and the weather were too tough for the young, inexperienced dogs, and it was unfair to have put them in that situation.

They had suffered: some had torn pads and broken claws and others frostbitten flanks. All were exhausted. Seppala swore he would never again abuse their trust in him, and he knew that in return for his loyalty, he would receive "their simple, canine faith"—a life-saving faith.

FOR THE rest of the spring and summer, Seppala nursed his dogs back to health. Then, in the fall, he began to train them again for the 1915 sweepstakes. Gradually, the dogs recovered their health and confidence. A few weeks before the race, Seppala took them over the trail and stashed hamburger meat in coal-oil cans he had set up at strategic points along the route. He switched the dogs to a high-protein diet of beef and mutton and had his brother, Asle, build him a racing sled which had extra long runners, so that he could better control the turns. He sewed racing harnesses for the animals. By the eve of the race, with all the preparations completed, he was so excited that "I felt like a loaded gun ready to explode any second."

That night, he had trouble sleeping. Despite every effort, he worried. He still had to rely on luck, on being in the right place and at the right time at the very moment the weather turned. He also had his main competitor Allan to worry about. By then Allan had won three sweepstakes.

On the morning of April 14, the racers lined up at the starting line for the eighth annual sweepstakes. With the drop of a flag, the teams burst across the line. Seppala, by contrast, started off at a leisurely pace, and word of his slow start immediately got back to the gamblers at the Board of Trade. Seppala wasn't worried. He knew his dogs well: they took their time to warm up, but they always finished strong, and he did not want to tire himself out too early. About sixty miles into the race he caught up with several drivers who had stopped at the Timber shelter cabin for a break. (Rest stops were not mandatory; it was up to the drivers to decide when and where they should stop.) He stayed long enough to wolf down a bowl of soup and a sandwich.

Several hours later, he caught up with Allan, who had stopped briefly at a cabin about one hundred miles from the start. Seppala passed the Scotsman, and ten miles down the trail he stopped where he had stashed the hamburger meat for the dogs. Soon afterwards, Allan was back in the race, and their game of cat-and-mouse began in earnest.

By the second day of the race, Seppala's team was setting a steady, rapid pace. He sensed they still had plenty of energy to burn, and at one point the dogs smelled reindeer and geared up for a long, sustained gallop, one of the fastest rides of Seppala's career.

At a shelter cabin 140 miles down the trail, Seppala joined his opponent for a bowl of soup. As he was getting ready to leave, a spectator came up to him and suggested he get some rest, but Seppala replied that he was out to beat the Scotsman and had to set off at once. On the way out, Allan looked up at him from his soup and "smiled back at me enigmatically. He and I both knew I was up against a tough job."

For the next thirty miles Seppala remained far out in the lead, with no sign of his opponent. Then, as he reached the top of the Divide, he "could see a team way back worming its way over the crooked trail, looking like a big reptile in the distance." The race was far from over. Thirty miles on, Seppala reached Candle, the turnaround point where he had hoped to get a brief rest. One of the dogs came loose during a judges' inspection and Seppala knew he would be disqualified if he did not catch the animal. He ran around after the dog and finally backed him up against the shouting crowd. Scared and confused, the dog bit Seppala's hand, but he still managed to catch him.

News of the injury soon flashed through to Nome: Seppala would have to drive the last 204 miles with just one hand, and the gamblers upped the odds against him. He had lost valuable time, and thirty miles out of Candle, while heading back up over the Divide, Allan passed him at a good speed.

But the Scotsman's show of strength may have been a bluff. Allan would often psych out his opponents by pretending his dogs were in top form, and Seppala did not take the bait. As Allan pulled away up the Divide, Seppala noticed that one of Allan's dogs looked tired and another had run loose behind the sled. Seppala pretended his team was tuckered out and let Allan pull even farther ahead. Then, when Allan was too far away to notice, he picked up the pace.

For much of the third day, Seppala continued to track Allan, staying a good half hour behind him. In a long-distance race, competitors would try to throw off the rest schedule of their opponents in the hopes of tiring them out. Seppala was determined to pressure Allan into making a mistake, but he was determined at the same time to run his own race. At one point, he stopped to rest at a cabin and let the young dogs rest in the sunshine. The dogs were quiet and relaxed, basking in the sun. It was the end of the day for them. Seppala had trouble getting them up. Only the leader was raring to go. Back at the cabin, a spectator misinterpreted the dogs' brief reverie and told the gamblers back in Nome that "Seppala's team is all in, and he can't even get them started."

Then he placed a $100 bet on Allan.

Seppala got the dogs back up and they were on track again. Death Valley was an easy ride for both drivers and each one sailed through the usually stormy valley with ease. Then, toward the end of the third day, Seppala pulled into Boston, about one hundred miles from the finish line. Allan, who had managed to keep a steady gap between them since the Divide, had arrived half an hour earlier. While their dogs rested outside, the two opponents sat at opposite ends of a table. Seppala told Allan that his dogs were tired out but that he was going to drive another twenty-six miles to Council. There, he said, he would take a long rest. Allan replied that his dogs were in excellent shape. He needed a few hours of rest in Boston and would then make the dash to Nome. He fully expected to cross the finish line before noon of the following day.

Seppala doubted Allan could do it. He had driven thirty miles more than Seppala that day and he badly needed a long rest. There were 106 miles to go before the finish line. Allan watched as Seppala got back on the sled. Again, the Norwegian's young Siberians seemed to be enjoying the sun and appeared reluctant to get back up. "They were dragging along slowly" out of Boston, Seppala recalled, "and to all appearances were pretty tired and not able to go many miles more; but I was banking on the Siberian traits I knew so well."

Sure enough, just outside the camp, a rabbit jumped on the trail and the dogs clicked into high gear and were soon running as if they were just starting the race. They kept up the pace all the way to the next planned stop, at Council. There, Seppala learned that Allan had left Boston after resting for four hours. The musher usually stayed for six hours at that spot. Allan was worried about his competition.

Seppala, meanwhile, bedded down for a full six hours of rest. The dogs would need it for the last eighty miles to Nome. Three hours into his light sleep, Seppala awoke at around ten-thirty to the sound of Allan's dogs arriving at the camp. The Scotsman lingered a few minutes and then drove on. Seppala panicked and began to gather his things and hook up the dogs. He had three of them on the line when, about thirty minutes later, Allan was back. The driver claimed that his leader had lost the way in the dark. Seppala wondered if this was a ruse to break his rest and get him back on the trail. But he remembered his pledge to run his own race and curled back up to sleep with the dogs.

Two hours later, he awoke and quietly hitched up the team. Lookouts working for Allan alerted the Scotsman, and twenty minutes after Seppala left Council, Allan was in hot pursuit. By the time Seppala reached the Timber shelter cabin twenty miles away, Allan had closed the gap to four minutes. Seppala picked up speed. He reached the coast and went up Topkok Mountain. At the top, he looked back and saw no sign of Allan. A thick fog hugged the midriff of the mountain. These were the last fifty miles, and here Allan would usually put on a burst of speed and topple the competition. Seppala began his descent from the windswept summit, struggling to keep the sled upright as it bounced over bumps in the fog. At the base of the mountain, the fog lifted and the team raced into the sunshine. Seppala looked over his shoulder, expecting to see "Scotty come dashing after me, emerging from the cloud down Topkok Mountain. But there was no sign of him."

Seppala traveled another twenty-two miles to the checkpoint at Port Safety and stopped long enough to ask spectators if they knew of his rival's whereabouts. Allan, they said, had only just arrived at Solomon, the checkpoint ten miles back. The four-minute gap between them had widened to forty-five. A little after 3:00 P.M., Seppala passed Fort Davis, where the cannon boomed at his approach, and a few minutes later he crossed the finish line. He was tired and shivering from the cold. It would be another two hours before Allan arrived.

Seppala's reputation was nearly secure.

FOR THE next two years, Seppala dominated the All Alaska Sweepstakes as well as other local races. What seemed to astound people most was his ability to get the most out of his dogs. It was almost uncanny, one competitor said. "That man is super-human. He passed me at least once on every day of the race and I was not loafing any. I couldn't see that he drove the dogs. He just clucked to them every now and then and they lay into their collars harder than I've ever seen dogs do it before.

"Something came out of him and went into those dogs with that clucking. You've heard of some men who hold an unnatural control over others—hypnotism, I guess you call it. I suppose it's just as likely to work on dogs, and Seppala certainly has it if anyone has."

In addition to preparing for the races, Seppala continued to earn his title by ferrying U.S. officials, Hammon employees, and an occasional accident victim across Alaska. On one occasion, he helped police chase down a criminal.

Seppala became a celebrity of sorts at the roadhouses, the log cabins that had sprung up along the trails to accommodate travelers. Awed patrons would help him harness the dogs and they would line up to watch him start out on the trail.

"I am proud of my racing trophies," Seppala once said, "but I would trade them all for the satisfaction of knowing that my dogs and I tried honestly to give our very best in humanitarian service to our fellowman, regardless of race, creed, color, in Alaska's pioneer days. Often the going was rough—sometimes my courage was greater than my team's—several times I was ready to quit but was ashamed because of the great fighting heart of the Siberian Husky."

NEARLY A decade after the last sweepstakes, with thousands of trail miles behind him, Seppala had a new lead dog, a Siberian Husky named Togo. At the age of twelve, the black and gray leader had become Seppala's favorite. The relationship was based on friendship as much as on partnership and mutual need. They were "inseparably linked," a friend said. "One does not speak of one without mention of the other." They would often romp together at night, and Seppala's favorite game was to try to grab Togo's feet while the dog danced. If Seppala was tired, he often sat by the fire with the dog next to him.

Togo simply seemed to know what to do, Seppala once told a reporter. One time, before the start of an eight-mile race, he had hitched the dog up to a sled driven by a young girl who had never ridden before, and he whispered in the dog's ear: "Go to it. I'll be waiting here for you."

Togo sped through the course and headed straight for Seppala, who was kneeling at the finish line. As the two rolled over and wrestled in the snow, a few spectators wiped tears from their eyes.

Now, as Seppala led the dogs through their drills in the Sawtooth Mountains, he felt lucky to have Togo with him for the round trip to Nulato. Togo had accompanied his master on every important journey, and together they had covered nearly 55,000 miles of trail. They had saved each other's lives many times crossing the frozen Norton Sound, and despite Togo's advanced age, Seppala still felt that wherever they went together, he traveled "with a sense of security."

This time there would be no cash prizes, no records set. They would be saving lives.

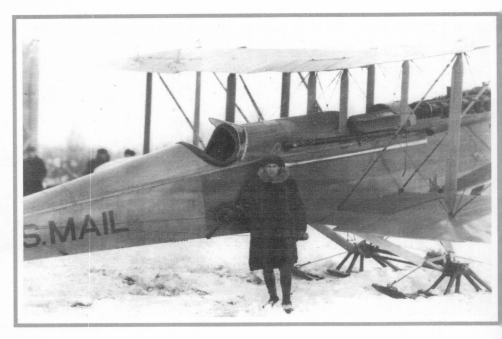

Aviator Carl Ben Eielson after completing the historic first air-mail flight in Alaska in February of 1924, an achievement many believed was the beginning of the end of dog driving in Alaska. (Anchorage Museum of History and Art/B72.88.44)

5

Flying Machines

"Diphtheria Rages in Nome; No Antitoxin; Remedy Sought by Plane on 50-Day Dog Trail."

— *The New York Times*, JANUARY 28, 1925

O N JANUARY 26, six days after the outbreak, on a bitterly cold Monday morning more than seven hundred miles northeast of Nome, a messenger from the local Signal Corps office knocked on the door of William Fentress Thompson's home on Eighth Avenue between Lacey and Noble streets in Fairbanks. Thompson, the publisher and editor of the *Fairbanks Daily News-Miner*, was barely out of bed when he took the urgent message:

Could aviator at Fairbanks put plane in commission within 48 hours to carry supply of antitoxin to Nome, for relief of diphtheria epidemic there? Answer quick, collect. Dan Sutherland, Alaskan delegate to U.S. Congress.

Thompson dressed quickly. This was the first he had heard of an epidemic, and his mind raced for a lead for his evening newspaper. Thompson was in his early sixties, had been a newspaperman on the frontier for most of his life, and was by now accustomed to risk. He was a stern-looking man, with a sharp, angular face, but his eyes gave away his true personality. They were almond-shaped and peered out from behind his round spectacles with the mischievous excitement of a child with his hand in the cookie jar. He never shied away from controversy, and made a point of standing his ground, a trait that had earned him his fair share of critics and the nickname "Wrong Font," a play on his first two initials and the printer's symbol for the wrong typeface. Throughout his career, Thompson had seen gold towns boom and bust across the Yukon Territory and Alaska as the easy gold ran out in the creeks and rivers and the miners fled. For the past decade he had watched his own town of Fairbanks teeter on the edge of a similar fate—one he was no longer willing to accept.

Built on the banks of the Chena River, a tributary of the Tanana, Fairbanks had been known as "the biggest log cabin city in the world" in the years following the discovery of gold in 1902. A bustling city and a main distribution point for the Interior, it linked the settlements with Alaska's ice-free ports to the south, first by trail and now by railroad. But as the placer gold diminished and the Interior villages emptied, the population of Fairbanks dwindled. World War I did further economic damage, and by 1925 the town was in a multi-year struggle to keep economic ruin at bay. So, by extension, was Thompson. His readership had been reduced by nearly half, and almost single-handedly he wrote, edited, and published each edition of the *News-Miner*. He made it his personal mission not only to inform readers but also to keep up their "flattened spirits," as one reader described. "Wrong Font" wrote about everything and anything, considering nothing too sacred or holy or political to be treated with his tabloid sensibility. He once expressed his disappointment with Fairbanks's children for not being mischievous enough on the eve of Halloween, and when the daughter of the chocolate manufacturer Ghirardelli died, the headline read: "Lost His Chocolate Drop."

Thompson practiced a sort of booster journalism. He hunted down and supported schemes he thought could bring money into the town—whether or not the community approved. He had been instrumental in building a flour mill and a farmer's bank to finance the development of the Tanana Valley's agriculture, but he had also rebelled against a town council decision to demolish the red light district. During the early years of Prohibition he had allegedly taken money from liquor interests to use his newspaper to promote drink-

ing. Certainly, Thompson enjoyed a drink and was a vocal enthusiast—liquor stores and bars generated cash.

By 1925, his hard work and hard living had begun to take their
toll. A year earlier he had sought medical attention outside the territory and returned in failing health. Thompson had been working and
betting hard for the past few years on another important scheme he
hoped would play a role in the town's salvation as well as his own: the
fledging business of the Fairbanks Airplane Corporation. With the
telegram in hand from the Alaskan delegate, he realized that a successful air rescue could energize the fledging airline and help lure
business back to town. Thompson was not a mere opportunist. He
had a sincere desire to help the people of Nome, and if he could
arrange a mercy mission, well, he would be doing all of Alaska a favor.

Thompson walked around the house with Sutherland's telegram.
It was 50 below zero outside and there were very few people on the
street. He reread the message as he considered the news from Nome
and all its implications. This would be his last great campaign.

OVER THE past three years, Thompson had become obsessed with
the development of an arctic airline industry. Since the end of World
War I the territory had become a beacon for former army pilots seek-
ing adventure, and in 1923 Thompson and a group of businessmen
formed the Farthest-North Airplane Company and hired a former
army pilot from North Dakota named Carl Ben Eielson.

Alaskan delegate Dan Sutherland had encouraged Eielson in 1922
to quit his job as a congressional guard in Washington, D.C., and
move to Fairbanks to take up piloting in the northern territory. The
two had spoken enthusiastically about the future of Alaskan flight,
and Sutherland soon found a temporary job for the pilot.

In Fairbanks, Eielson became fast friends with Thompson. They
would stay up late in the publisher's cluttered office, "drinking homebrew and talking aviation." Together, they persuaded a banker, Dick
Wood, to put up money for a plane, and they soon had sufficient
funds to build a crude runway, a 1,200-foot-long, 600-foot-wide

stump-ridden strip at one end of the local baseball field. It was good enough, and by the summer of 1923 Eielson was flying passengers on the company's single airplane, a Curtiss-built "Jenny." Just a few months later Farthest-North Airplane merged with its only rival, the Alaska Aerial Transportation Company, founded by a senior conductor of the railroad. The company was renamed the Fairbanks Airplane Corporation.

The company now had three planes and two pilots, Eielson and a former barnstormer named Noel Wien. It was barely an airline, but the aircraft were up and flying, and they were the only ones in Alaska. Business was good in 1923 and 1924; the company flew everything from gold to supplies, and it ferried passengers from one city to the next. With few exceptions, everything arrived safely.

The two pilots quickly built up reputations as courageous and capable men. Wien became the first pilot in North America to fly north of the Arctic Circle, and in February 1924, Eielson made the first winter flight in Alaska, a 260-mile trip from Fairbanks to McGrath on one of ten experimental air-mail runs scheduled by the U.S. Post Office for that winter. On two of those runs a makeshift flying ambulance had been set up and Eielson transported two patients back to the hospital in Fairbanks. Thompson had great faith in the company's future.

About a month before the Nome epidemic broke out, Fairbanks Airplane sold approximately $15,000 worth of stock to raise money for a fourth and much larger plane, an eight-passenger aircraft with an enclosed cabin. At Thompson's urging, dozens of Fairbanks residents bought stakes in the company. Among those investors was Sutherland.

Fairbanks lies midway between Tokyo and New York, and many then believed that a new air route across the Arctic to Asia could establish the Interior town as the "crossroads city of the world." This was not a far-fetched idea in 1925; five years earlier, the U.S. Army Air Service had organized a joint flight of four planes from New York to Nome and back as a demonstration of long-distance travel and a clear illustration of the safety of the northern skies. The De Havilland biplane bombers, known as the Black Wolf Squadron because of the insignia painted on the fuselage, took off from Mitchell Field, Long Island, on July 15, 1920, and flew north to Canada and British Columbia, then across Alaska to Fairbanks, making fourteen stops. From there, they tracked the Tanana and Yukon rivers, and three hours later landed safely on a sandbar in the small town of Ruby. The weather was bad, and the four pilots were forced to lay over for two days before taking off for Nulato, further west down the Yukon River. Then they banked to the north over the mountains and made a bee-line for Nome. Low cloud cover forced the planes down to 2,500 feet, barely above the snow-capped peaks, and when they emerged over the Bering Sea coast, early squalls began to batter them. They flew through heavy snow all the way to Nome. A little over three hours after taking off from Ruby, the Black Wolf Squadron landed at the old parade grounds at Fort Davis.

All of Nome had come out to watch. For days the town had been busy laying out a landing strip by widening and straightening the curved road at the old army fort. Welch and his nurses came, just in case there was an accident, and Seppala arrived with some of his dogs to look at the competition. Seppala was intrigued by the new technology and asked whether he could climb up into one of the cockpits "to try it on for size."

The New York–to–Nome round-trip flight—a trip of more than 9,000 miles—was proof positive that long-distance aerial transportation was possible in the far north, and Thompson was now convinced that Nome could be saved with a single flight out of Fairbanks. All they needed was a pilot. And this was a problem. Eielson was in Washington trying to lobby the government to develop northern flight and authorize permanent air mail, and Wien had gone in search of the company's new aerial limousine.

Thompson began to consider other options. He remembered that just a few days earlier he had met a Justice Department agent named Roy Darling who was in Fairbanks on business. The special investigator seemed like an even-tempered and responsible fellow, and Thompson remembered that he had flying experience.

Before joining the Justice Department, the thirty-eight-year-old Darling had learned to fly and handle weaponry at the Royal Aeronautical School and the Royal School of Infantry in Canada, and he subsequently joined the U.S. Navy as an ordnance specialist in 1917. He was based at the Indian Head proving grounds in Maryland, where he had tested guns, bombs, and other weapons for the navy. It was clear that he was officer material: his superiors described him as "cheerful, forceful, active, and painstaking," and he was made a senior lieutenant.

But his career had been cut short in May 1919. While en route from Washington, D.C., to Indian Head, the seaplane in which he was traveling malfunctioned and plunged 500 feet into the water. Darling broke his right femur, fractured his jaw, lacerated his lower lip, and broke the arches on both feet. A series of operations had left him with one leg shorter than the other and a severe limp. He was forced to walk with a cane, wore an elevator shoe, and had a very limited range of motion in one of his knees. His feet hurt and he often felt stiff; to make matters worse, many of his teeth had been broken or pushed askew and he chewed his food with difficulty.

With his severe limp and his scarred face, Darling cut a relatively rugged figure, even by Alaskan standards. Courage and stoicism were much admired in the territory, as was a measure of self-sacrifice. Thompson did not fail to notice that this remade man, wounds and all, might just be the one for the job. He was tough and daring. From the point of view of an inveterate newshound like Thompson, Darling was the mother lode, a made-to-order hero.

THOMPSON TOO had a bad leg from an old accident, and he picked up his cane as soon as he finished his coffee and hobbled across the frozen town to see the "broken flyer." Darling was still in bed, so Thompson sat him up, plied him with coffee, and began to tell him the whole, sad story about Nome's children. It didn't take long to convince the man: despite his accident six years earlier, Darling was eager to fly.

There were a few conditions, Darling explained. He would have to agree to keep the news from his wife, Caroline, who had settled into a new home in Anchorage, and he had to get permission from the Justice Department. He would also need clearance from the U.S. Navy so that if he crashed, Caroline would be eligible for benefits. (Darling was technically on medical leave from the navy because of his injuries, and he was not due for official retirement with honors and benefits until June 1925.)

Darling was ready to go to Nome even if he "had to go hanging onto the tail of a kite." So Thompson asked him to go across town to examine the three planes stored in Stewart's warehouse and report back.

Early that afternoon, Darling walked over to Third Avenue with a mechanic named Farnsworth and another man, Fred Struthers, the manager of Fairbanks Airplane, and the three of them rolled open the heavy doors of the warehouse. It was nearly dark. One of them turned on the flashlight they had borrowed from Smith's Hardware & Gun Store down the street. In the middle of the drafty warehouse they saw the two dilapidated airships, surplus training planes from World War I. There was a third old plane outside, and it was hardly in better shape.

The aircraft had been sitting in the makeshift hangar ever since the flying season ended in October, and their wings had been dismantled. The fabric coverings, which had once stretched taut over the wooden frames, had become weak from all the rough landings and the wind and rain. Dirt and oil caked the engines and propellers like a second skin, and the control wires for the rudders and elevators were draped along the sides of the fuselage. The machines had been badly in need of an overhaul even before they were stored away last fall.

The men examined each plane and agreed there was only one fit for the job. It was the *Anchorage*, a World War I surplus Standard J-1 biplane previously used to train army pilots. Its name was stenciled in red and black letters on the fuselage and its tail still carried the faded red, white, and blue insignia of the Army Air Service. The engine looked to be in fairly good shape; there was even an extra 30-gallon tank welded beneath the center of the uppermost wing. The *Anchorage* had been refitted with a 150-horsepower Hispano-Suiza engine, a fast and compact machine developed by a French automobile racer and used by combat pilots during the war. The moving parts, which included its drive shafts and overhead cams, had customized covers and were well protected from oil and dust. This was considered a great advantage in Alaska, where pilots would often use sandbars and marshes as impromptu landing strips.

The tank had been added the previous summer for the historic first flight between Anchorage and Fairbanks. Wien had been at the controls for the entire 350-mile route, but was so unfamiliar with the route that he decided to follow the railroad tracks all the way to Fairbanks. While flying over a series of forest fires, his vision was obscured by black smoke and he came perilously close to losing his way. He narrowly escaped death when a trestle suddenly loomed up out of the smoke. But a miss was as good as a mile, and in the end, the company decided that the flight had been a great success.

With the inspection over, Struthers, Farnsworth, and Darling shut the warehouse doors and walked over to Thompson's office to give him a complete report. The office was a small, cramped space with cases of lead type strewn among pieces of heavy printing equipment. There were no storm windows or double doors, and whenever someone entered the steam-heated room an icy fog rushed in behind them.

The *Anchorage* could be put back in flying shape and would be ready to "hit the air for Nome, rain or shine" within three days, the men told Thompson. The flight itself would take no more than six hours. It was all Thompson needed to hear. When they left, he headed for his desk. Above it was a framed copy of his Michigan high school paper, *The Howard City Snorter*. He began to type and did not look up until he was finished. A few hours later, Thompson had his story.

That evening, the *News-Miner* carried the tale of Nome's plight. It read like a rallying cry for help and featured Roy Darling, whom Thompson had described as Nome's "Forlorn Hope."

"The atmosphere is not right for flying, no flier would fly on a bet on such days as these. . . . EVERYTHING IS AGAINST the 'game,'" the lead story in the paper shouted. "Yet the emergency undoubtedly exists, and Fairbanks [is] in the eyes of the Flying World, and Nome is our neighbor and our pal. What you goin' to do? The answer is GO."

Before calling it a night, Thompson sent word of the plane's condition to Sutherland and asked him to get official permission for Darling to fly. Then in a telegram to Nome he proposed that the town "be of good cheer . . . the aviators are all gone at present . . . but if Washington will release Detective Darling now here on official business . . . [he] is 'rarin to go' to Nome's help. Have wired Washington accordingly. Nome can depend on Fairbanks to bring help or somebody will die trying."

MORE THAN 3,000 miles away in Washington, D.C., Dan Sutherland went to work. A supporter of home rule for Alaska and an advocate for breaking the West Coast's grip on the territory's lucrative fishing, shipping, mining, and lumber industries, Sutherland was a scrapper. He had recently startled Washington by appearing in the center of the business district in his suspenders, wearing neither coat nor vest. "I am allowing the dust of Washington to blow off me," he told a reporter, "so that I will be in finer trim to go after the gentlemen who are looting Alaska of its salmon and timber, and get quicker results when Congress convenes again." His persistence on Capitol Hill had earned him the nickname "Fighting Dan" back home.

Sutherland had a personal stake in Nome. He had been one of the first to step foot on its beach in the summer of 1900, having traveled aboard a whaler that crashed through the melting ice to beat the thousands of prospectors close behind. When the others left, he stayed on as a miner and part owner of one of Nome's freight companies. He knew the Alaskan winters well. When he turned to politics in his late thirties, he stumped thousands of miles accross the Interior on foot and by dogsled to win a seat on Alaska's first legislature after it became a territory in 1912. He was a popular representative, and in 1921 Alaskans voted him to be the territory's congressional delegate in Washington, D.C.

Soon after receiving Thompson's message, the now fifty-five-year-old delegate approached the Public Health Service and its chief, Hugh Cumming, the U.S. Surgeon General, and told him that Fairbanks was prepared to launch an unprecedented air rescue of Nome. A single flight would take just a few hours, Sutherland said, but a dogsled would take weeks. By then, many children would be dead.

Cumming listened carefully and told Sutherland he was open to the idea, whereupon Sutherland immediately cabled Mayor Maynard in Nome:

> Health Department will take immediate action to relieve the conditions at Nome. They are trying to get an airplane. Will keep you advised.

SUTHERLAND'S OTHER telegram, to Thompson, earlier that Monday morning, had been triggered by a wonderful discovery. The day before, a fifty-three-year-old doctor in the town of Anchorage had come across a supply of 300,000 units of antitoxin. Dr. John Bradley Beeson, chief surgeon of the Anchorage Railroad Hospital, had heard about Nome's epidemic and taken immediate action. He headed straight for the Signal Corps office next to the railroad tracks and fired off a telegram to Alaska's governor, Scott C. Bone:

> 300,000 units of serum located in railway hospital here . . . package can be shipped by train to Nenana. . . . Could serum be carried to Nome by mail drivers and dog teams?

At about the same time, the Public Health Service had found 1.1 million units of antitoxin in various hospitals along the West Coast, and these had been ordered sent to Seattle where they could be forwarded to Alaska. But the next available ship north, the *Alameda*, was still out at sea and would not dock until Saturday, January 31, several days away. Worse still, the boat would take between six and seven days to reach the port at Seward, and by the time the serum had made its way to Nome, many more children would be dead.

Beeson's serum would have a two-week head start. Although it was not sufficient to wipe out the epidemic, it could keep it in check for a while longer.

Governor Bone directed Beeson to prepare the serum at once and send it north to the Interior by train. In the twelve hours it took for the serum to reach the Interior, he would decide whether to allow an airplane rescue or to rely on the dogs.

Beeson was a competent and capable doctor, and he had become somewhat of a celebrity in Alaska. Four years earlier, he had been in the local papers after a house call of more than five hundred miles to the small town of Iditarod, where a banker was in urgent need of treatment. An impromptu relay of dog teams was set up along the route to carry Beeson to the Interior gold town, and they traveled at such speed and over such rough terrain that the drivers had to lash the doctor onto the sled.

At one point, the sled had broken through the ice and Beeson was plunged into the water. His hands were too cold to untie the knots and he struggled to free himself. He felt the sled lurch. He could see up through the surface of the water and so was a witness to his own rescue as the dogs skillfully pulled the sled safely onto the bank. There were other mishaps along the route: one of the drivers' toes froze and another driver was hurt, and Beeson had had to drive a sled for the very first time.

In retrospect, he was astonished he had made it all the way, and equally surprised that his patient was still alive when he arrived. The patient's name was Claude Baker, and he was already in the advanced stages of pulmonary tuberculosis. There was little Beeson could do but try to get him back to Anchorage, where he could receive round-the-clock care.

Unable to set up a relay for the return journey, Beeson set off with one driver and little hope. By fortunate coincidence, he met up along the route with Leonhard Seppala, who was headed to Anchorage with two officials of the Alaska Road Commission. Seppala was traveling with four teams and forty-three dogs, and he agreed to break away with Beeson and his patient. Seppala was fast and he drove a strong team. They climbed over a 150-foot-high glacier and careened down a steep grade of glare ice and up over Rainey Pass. About 150 miles west of Anchorage the snow began to fall and Seppala had to break trail ahead of the dogs, but they made it back to the hospital without incident.

Beeson's house call had taken a month from beginning to end.

Now, as Beeson looked over the amber-colored glass vials of serum on the main floor of Anchorage's four-story hospital, he recalled every mile of that unbearably cold trip, and each jolt of the sled. If the shipment had to be carried by dog team all the way to Nome, it would need protection, so Beeson padded the inside of a container and placed the vials inside. He took a heavy quilt and wrapped it around the container, then placed it into a wooden crate, covering it with thick brown cloth. When he was done, he pinned a note to the cloth instructing whoever would be carrying the serum to warm the container up for fifteen minutes after each stop on the trail. By the time he was through, the package weighed 20 pounds.

Beeson carried the serum over to the railway station where the locomotive stood by and handed the package to the conductor, Frank Knight. Knight placed it in a snug corner of the baggage car. As the engineer blew the whistle, the train jolted forward. Beeson sent a message to Governor Bone telling him the serum would be arriving in Nenana by the following night, Tuesday, January 27.

"Appreciate your prompt action for Nome relief," Bone replied.

BACK IN his office, Bone considered his options. The decision would be his whether to send the serum by dog team or by plane. With his slight paunch and bushy gray eyebrows, the sixty-four-year-old governor had a kind and warm way about him. He made friends easily, and was relatively broad-minded. Bone's trajectory to the governorship had been unusual: he had been a journalist most of his life and worked his way up the pressroom ranks to become editor of the *Seattle Post-Intelligencer*.

As the gateway to Alaska, Seattle was home to a number of West Coast businesses that had control of a large part of the state's principal industries, including commercial fishing, lumber, and shipping, and Bone had begun to take an interest in the territory while working at the paper. In 1913, in his capacity as editor, he had been invited to tour the territory with the Alaskan Bureau of the Seattle Chamber of Commerce, and he and several others had traveled the length of the territory, visiting nearly every major town, including Nome. Less than ten years later, after a brief time as publicity director for the Republican National Committee, in 1921, he became the tenth governor of Alaska.

The governorship, a position appointed by the U.S. president, was a tough and in many ways a thankless job. The salary was a pittance; a previous governor had once complained that he spent $10,000 annually in office, $3,000 more than he was earning. Many Alaskans resented the fact that they did not even have the right to elect their own leader, and some viewed the position as a branch of the meddlesome federal government.

While Bone may have been the highest official in a region more than twice the size of Texas, he exercised little executive control. Most decisions about the territory's development, the allocation of resources and taxes, were in the hands of conflicting and often uninformed bureaucrats in Washington.

For nearly every decision, Bone had to wade through a swamp of federal bureaucracy, a situation that had become familiar to every governor before him. A case in point: neither Bone nor the taxpayers of Alaska had the authority to move the governor's modest office without Washington's approval.

Since 1906, when the capital of Alaska had finally moved to Juneau from the former Russian outpost of Sitka on one of the islands of the Inside Passage, each one of Alaska's governors had been forced to work out of a cramped and dilapidated log cabin. By 1924, the two-story cabin was in such a state of disrepair that both floors slanted and the ground floor rested on steam pipes. An architect authorized by the Interior Department at Bone's urgent behest reported that the crumbling cabin was "unfit for habitation" and warned the governor to move out before winter, for it could easily catch fire or get swept away by a strong wind.

Washington continued its indecision until the day the architect's prophecy came true. On January 5, 1925, the floor in the center of the building settled on the boiler and burst into flames.

Bone was not the only Alaskan official frustrated by the federal bureaucracy. "It will not be long," one Alaskan lawyer quipped at the time, "before Alaska will need a license signed by a cabinet officer to kill a mosquito."

Nearly six decades after its purchase by the United States, Alaska still could not legally determine its own fate, and it would be another thirty-four years before it received statehood. It was run by at least thirty-eight federal bureaus and five cabinet officers who were all—as Bone wrote in one of his articles for the *Saturday Evening Post*—"interlocked, overlapped, cumbersome and confusing, each intent upon its own particular business, jealous of its own success and prerogatives, and all more or less unrelated and independent in their operations."

Bone often used his pen to rail against the red tape, which he said maimed the pioneer spirit of Alaska, and to educate Americans about "The Land that Uncle Sam Bought and then Forgot," the headline of an article he had written for the *Review of Reviews*.

By 1925, Bone was fed up and determined to leave the territory for good by mid-year. "No one understands Alaska," the frustrated governor had once told a reporter while on a trip to Washington. "Even official Washington does not understand what we have. They wire me to step over to Nome to look up a little matter, not realizing that it takes me 11 days to get there."

Bone knew that the issue of transporting the serum could get bogged down in red tape and become a political football. Delegate Sutherland and *News-Miner* editor Thompson were pushing hard for an air rescue, and while Bone leaned toward the idea, he wanted to make sure that his was a responsible choice. The final decision was his alone, and no amount of pressure, political or otherwise, could sway him.

Bone was familiar with the debate surrounding the potential for an Alaskan airline industry, and he had no doubt that air routes would play an important role in the territory's future. In 1923, when Warren Harding became the first U.S. president to visit Alaska, Bone was among a crowd who watched Eielson fly over Nenana in his biplane and perform loops, spirals, and stalls in the president's honor. Harding was in town to celebrate the completion of the railway line, and as Bone watched the president drive a golden spike into the tracks, he may have already known that the future was in the skies above them.

Still, Bone began to question the mercy flight to Nome.

The weather—one of the most crucial factors in almost every aspect of Alaskan life—had turned bitterly cold, and most travel within the territory was at a near standstill. For over a week, a continental arctic high-pressure system had pushed temperatures in the Interior to their lowest levels in nearly twenty years. Because the Interior was a basinlike stretch of land surrounded by mountains and high hills, it was difficult for a competing warmer weather system to blow in and dissipate the cold. And the cold grew deeper as the days wore on, stealing what little solar heat had been stored in the ground. No wonder the territory was known as "Seward's Ice Box," after Secretary of State William Henry Seward, who had bought the territory from the Russians in 1867.

The recent cold temperatures in the Interior had been front-page news in nearly every local newspaper. In Fairbanks, the post office had to shut down because there was not enough heat to keep the employees warm. Farther to the east in Canada's Yukon Territory, temperatures of minus 70 degrees forced a halt to the delivery of water and mail in Mayo and in Dawson City.

Meanwhile, an entirely different system was harassing Juneau and the other towns of southeastern Alaska, often called the Panhandle. In January, the temperature on average is close to freezing, relatively warm when compared to the Interior, but the amount of snowfall is high and the storms from the Gulf of Alaska frequent. From his new offices in the Goldstein Building—by far the tallest in Juneau—Bone could see the town digging out from beneath a snowstorm as 25-mile-per-hour winds whipped down the streets, creating 10-foot high drifts and traffic jams of cars and horse-drawn buggies.

The snowstorms and gales over the past several days had also created havoc in the shipping lanes. The steamer *Admiral Watson* limped down the Gastineau Channel into port that morning, listing dangerously from the layers of ice that coated its pilothouse, rails, and bow. It had been the stormiest voyage in memory, "an almost continuous succession of snowstorms and gales," the captain remembered.

Four days earlier, in the middle of an equally alarming weather system, the steamship *Alameda* had arrived with 400 tons of copper ore and cured herring. The ship had taken forty-eight hours to cross the Gulf of Alaska and its ninety passengers had been "shaken up by the rough passage," which was probably an understatement. Even during relatively calm voyages, the tall, narrow, and top-heavy *Alameda* "rolled like an old-fashioned churn. . . . "

"Just as she seemed to be lying almost flat on her side, she'd right herself with a shiver and come slowly back to an upright position, only to roll over just as far to the other side," one passenger recalled.

If strong winds and temperatures of 10 degrees above zero could do such damage to the two stalwarts of the Seattle-to-Juneau service, one could only imagine the dangers of flying a plane during an Alaskan storm.

The three aircraft in Fairbanks each had open cockpits, and Bone questioned whether any pilot, let alone an injured man like Darling, could survive any flight in temperatures of minus 50 degrees.

Until now, most flights in Alaska had taken place during the summer or in the warmer winter months. Eielson's experimental air-mail runs had been a success, but he had never flown in temperatures colder than minus 10 degrees—40 degrees warmer than the temperatures in Fairbanks that week.

Eielson had had to wear two pairs of heavy woolen socks, caribou-skin socks, a pair of moccasins that reached over his knees, a suit of heavy underwear, khaki breeches, heavy trousers of Hudson Bay duffle, a heavy shirt, sweater, marten-skin cap, goggles, and over all of that a reindeer-skin parka that went down to his knees and a hood trimmed with wolverine fur. He could barely climb into the plane, and in addition to the stacks of mail, he carried a full set of emergency gear just in case he crashed or became lost en route. He also carried tools, a sheepskin sleeping bag, ten days' worth of food, 5 gallons of oil, snowshoes, a gun, an ax, and repair materials, although he never had occasion to use them.

Eielson had crash-landed a few times, coming close to destroying his plane, but he had been lucky, all in all. Returning to Fairbanks on the first run, night fell and he got lost. Volunteers built a huge bonfire on the baseball field, wondering if the worst had occurred. Several hours later, they heard the sound of his motor in the distance. It was so dark by that time that they could hear the plane but could not see its wings until it "came within the rays of the bonfire." It was a near catastrophe. As Eielson landed, he had to guess where the front edge of the field was, misjudged, and broke off one of his skis on the top of a tree. When the plane hit the ground, it flipped forward on its nose and the propeller was crushed. The waiting crowd rushed to the plane to find Eielson shaken but otherwise all right. "We found him grinning behind the stick," one witness said, "but he was so stiff with cold and exhaustion that we had to lift him out of the cockpit."

On his final mail run, Eielson encountered a patch of mud on the airstrip, causing the plane to nose over once again, breaking the propeller, rudder, and wing struts. Eielson rolled out, then released the straps on a passenger he'd agreed to take back with him, dropping him haplessly but harmlessly on his head.

In the course of the mail runs, during which he'd spent fewer than fifty hours in the air, Eielson had gone through a large crate of spare parts, and the U.S. Post Office refused to send more. With none available in Fairbanks, the Post Office called a halt to the two remaining runs. Of the ten scheduled runs, Eielson completed eight.

Despite the crash landings, Eielson's flights had become famous. In a cabinet meeting in Washington, someone had read out an account of Eielson's adventure, and the story so captured the imagination of President Calvin Coolidge that he sent Eielson a congratulatory note.

U.S. Post Office officials, however, felt the territory was not yet ready for a regular air-mail service, and they asked for their crippled plane back. In a letter to Eielson, Assistant Postmaster General Paul Henderson told him in no uncertain terms that they had considered the experiment only a partial success: "There are many things which must be done before we can continue on a permanent basis our use of the airplane in mail carrying in Alaska," Henderson wrote. But he promised he would consider trying again at some future date.

Eielson had been flying a government-issue De Havilland, a plane that had once been considered the workhorse of the mail service and that had also been used during wartime as a bomber and a reconnaissance craft. The De Havilland was far sturdier than the flimsy biplanes owned by Fairbanks Airplane.

Even if Thompson's "Forlorn Hope" could overcome the wind, the cold, and the mechanical limitations of the time, there was one factor that Thompson, Dan Sutherland, and Mayor Maynard were overlooking. The days were shorter in January, and Darling would have a limited number of daylight hours in which to fly safely. Flying at night was a risky proposition. The U.S. Post Office did not make a serious attempt until 1923, on the Chicago-to-Cheyenne segment of its Transcontinental Air Mail Route, where officials made elaborate preparations on the ground as well as in midair. They installed revolving beacons that could be seen for 150 miles. Built on 50-foot towers, these became "lighthouses in the sky." The beacons were placed in five cities along the air-mail route, and between them, the Post Office laid out emergency landing fields, illuminated by smaller, less powerful beacons. As an extra precaution to aid pilots, flashing ground lights fueled by acetylene were placed every three miles between the emergency landing fields. The planes were also fitted with state-of-the-art technology, including wing tips with lights, and cockpits with radio transmitters to alert the pilots to bad weather ahead.

The old biplane *Anchorage*, by comparison, had no navigational tools save for a magnetic compass, which had proven to be unreliable. Any pilot taking off from Fairbanks for Nome would find himself in the dark, in every sense, without a light to guide him along the route or a radio to warn him of an approaching blizzard.

To make matters worse, the territory had been mapped out in haphazard fashion. When the Post Office and other territorial officials organized the experimental mail runs in 1924, they had to consult three maps because each one showed a different topographical outline of the route. The pilots thus learned the terrain the hard way. A mountain measuring 1,000 feet on a map would loom up at 5,000 feet, and a riverbank that might have been considered as an emergency landing spot would turn out to be a tiny creek in the middle of a forest.

An Alaskan pilot had to be fearless and he was often forced to rely on instinct. Wien once landed on top of a 300-foot hill in the Interior to pick up a sick man, then found to his horror that he had insufficient room for takeoff. Wien "jumped off" the mountain in the hope that the light plane would catch a lift from the wind. Again, he'd been lucky.

Landings and takeoffs were the worst: the Standard J-1 biplanes like *Anchorage* and other planes of the era had no brakes and had to drag to a stop by means of a single skid on the bottom of the tail. Baseball fields, marshes, and riverbanks all served as airfields. Not until the late 1930s would federal funds be set aside for safe fields and organized air routes in Alaska. Until then, the average plane was expected to crash twice or even three times a year.

And even if Darling made it across the Interior, all the daring in the world could not help him up the Bering Sea coast. He knew none of the local landmarks—the big rock of Besboro Island off the coast of Unalakleet, the lopsided shape of Topkok Mountain east of Cape Nome—signposts that might have helped guide him in the event a gale blew him off course and out over the ice.

Later pilots traveling over the coast often found themselves flying into hazy skies that appeared to blend into the ice and snow below.

The result was a bewildering panorama that, from the vantage point of the cockpit, was like "flying inside a milk bottle," a void without reference points. A pilot could barely tell whether he was flying straight up or if he had been inverted or gone into a spin. Further, it would be difficult for any plane, let alone the *Anchorage*, to survive the coast's sudden snowstorms and heavy gusts, which could be as powerful as 75 mph.

"Airplanes can't fly into 60 mph winds," Wien once remarked of the fleet in Fairbanks after he had battled for hours against a headwind that eventually forced him down.

Anchorage's engine, while a model of modernity by the standards of the early 1920s, was like any other motor of its time—cooled by water and therefore unreliable in severe cold. Antifreeze had not yet been invented and pilots had experimented, with limited success, with various mixtures of alcohol. (Prestone coolants, or ethylene glycol, were not introduced until 1931.) Further, the oil turned viscous at about 10 degrees above zero, and whenever a pilot landed, he would have to set up a fire pot beneath the engine to keep it warm while the passenger or a local mechanic drained the oil into a pan and warmed it over the coals.

Water-cooled engines shook so hard in the air in those days that bolts and screws would sometimes come loose. Water lines were broken, radiators were loosened, steam spouted from cracks, and spark plugs fouled. The engines sputtered and cut out, and the quiet, eerie hum of the wind through the guy wires would suddenly replace the roar of the engine. When air-cooled radial motors were introduced in 1926, the number of forced landings dropped by 25 percent.

In the 1920s, an engine failure usually meant death or, at the very least, serious injury. If a plane lost flying speed, it would go into a tailspin followed by an uncontrolled dive, and if the engine remained idle, there would be no possibility of recovery. It would be several years before the engineers would discover that a tailspin could be avoided by mounting sliding panels along the edge of the wings. When the plane tilted, the panels would slip forward and smooth out the airflow.

The aircraft had hardly been designed with arctic travel in mind, and the army did not even begin to perform systematic experiments in extreme temperatures until the 1930s.

There were other potential dangers as well. Snow and ice could clog the air filters and inlet connections, thus starving the carburetor of the oxygen needed for combustion; many a plane was forced to the ground when ice gathered on the radiators, propeller hubs, and wings—deicing technology still lay in the future.

EIELSON WOULD become one of the first pilots to master an engine in minus-40-degree weather. In April 1928, while flying over Point Barrow, north of Nome, the extreme cold caused the engine to falter repeatedly. To keep it operating, Eielson went into a steep climb above the clouds where the sun's rays warmed the engine. He repeated the procedure every twenty minutes for over two hours. The procedure worked but he had nearly run out of gas.[1]

The dream of northern flight was not exclusive to Thompson, Sutherland, and Eielson. Explorers had envisaged conquering the Arctic and Antarctic by balloon, dirigible, or plane for at least two decades. After his successful bid by dog sled to the North Pole in 1909, Robert Peary predicted that the Arctic would be "reconnoitered and explored through the air." Roald Amundsen learned to fly and earned his pilot's license less than a year after reaching the South Pole in 1911. Dog teams, while reliable, were slow and cumbersome. On one of his dog sled expeditions across the arctic ice pack in 1915, Vilhalmur Stefansson told a colleague that in the future a plane might cover in one day as much territory as a dog team could in a year.

In the 1920s, there were still thousands of square miles of Arctic Ocean that remained unseen. Many believed that unmapped islands

---

1. On November 9, 1929, Eielson and his mechanic Earl Borland disappeared while making a relief flight to bring out the cargo of the fur ship *Nanuk*, trapped in the ice off North Cape, Siberia. The wreckage from his plane was found on January 27, 1930, ninety miles from where the ship had been trapped. The crash was probably caused by bad weather and a broken altimeter.

existed, and some spoke of an uncharted continent in the icy wilderness between Spitsbergen, in Norway, and Alaska. These mythical territories possibly contained mineral wealth and could have strategic military value, given their location at the top of the world. Tidal studies pointed to the existence of such land. In the nineteenth and early twentieth centuries, whalers and explorers who had sailed up through the Bering Strait claimed to have seen a landmass north of Alaska. Peary, while traveling along the northern coast in Canada, reported snow-capped peaks far off in the distance to the northwest. (All of the sightings were later proven to be mirages, common to the Arctic.)

In the spring of 1923, Amundsen made the first attempt to fly to the polar rim, from Wainwright, near Point Barrow, Alaska, to Spitsbergen. The attempt ended in failure: Amundsen's Junkers J-13 metal monoplane crashed on a test flight after landing on the rough arctic ice. Several months later, in 1924, the U.S. Navy had planned to survey the area with its first rigid dirigible, the *Shenandoah*. Six planes were to accompany the balloon from Teller, about seventy miles north of Nome, but the navy called the expedition off at the last minute: it was too expensive and dangerous.

IT WAS clear to Governor Bone that flying to Nome would be a hazardous undertaking. In his opinion, the equipment was inadequate to handle the rigors of the northern winter, and although Darling had a deep supply of courage, he lacked the necessary experience. If he went down, the serum would go down with him, and so would Nome's chance to fight the epidemic.

On the other hand, a mail drive was not without risks. If Bone were to trace the mail trail from Nenana to Nome on a map, his finger would follow the course of the Tanana River to the point where it converged with the Yukon, 137 miles to the west at the village of Tanana. It would continue on or along the river for another 230 miles to the village of Kaltag, then over coastal mountains to the Bering Sea and up the coast to Nome.

The Tanana and Yukon rivers cut through the heart of the Interior, a land Jack London once described as a "pitiless" expanse of "the bright White Silence." One could travel for days in the Interior and never see another soul. "Nature has many tricks wherewith she convinces man of his finity," London wrote in his short story "The White Silence," but ". . . The most tremendous, the most stupefying of all, is the passive phase of the White Silence. All movement ceases, the sky clears, the heavens are as brass; the slightest whisper seems sacrilege, and man becomes timid, affrighted at the sound of his own voice. Sole speck of life journeying across the ghostly wastes of a dead world, he trembles at his audacity, realizes that his is a maggot's life, nothing more."

From Kaltag, the trail left the Yukon River and rose into the mountains and along a ninety-mile portage of plateau, forest, and river that tumbled out at the Bering Sea coast. The coast was often stormy and treacherous and, compared to the deep cold and nearly windless Interior, it offered an entirely different riding experience. The snow was icy and hard, the wind blew unimpeded for miles, and there were few trees to dip behind for protection or to cut down for fuel.

The trail followed the coast of the Bering Sea along Norton Sound for 208 miles, and traveled across its shifting fields of ice. It traversed lagoons and river deltas and passed through "blowholes" or wind tunnels. There was nowhere to hide along the coast during a blizzard or a gale, so drivers holed up in roadhouses whenever they could find one. When they could not, they would huddle behind a pressure ridge, ice hummock or boulder, and absent any natural protection, they made do with climbing into the sled.

In sum, the 674 miles between Nenana and Nome held every kind of danger. A driver caught unaware or without sufficient preparation risked serious injury or death.

Many parts of the trail were originally used by Natives for travel between summer and winter camps. It is estimated that the Kaltag portage had been used for centuries as a winter trade route between the Athabaskan Indians in the Interior and the Eskimos on the coast. When the Russian fur traders arrived in the late eighteenth century followed years later by an army of miners, the trails were expanded and served the white-owned trading and military posts and towns. As European settlers set up the telegraph lines and mail services along the trails, entrepreneurs set up roadhouses for travelers.

These roadhouses were the rough equivalent of small inns, simple log cabins insulated with mud and moss, or in the more remote areas, just a canvas tent with a large barrel stove. On the more popular trails, they were separated by about a day's travel, or a distance of about thirty to fifty miles, and provided a modest place to rest, eat, and warm up. Meals generally cost between one and two dollars, and wild game—whatever the proprietor could hunt or buy—was often the specialty of the week. There was freshly baked bread and local vegetables, and if a traveler was lucky he could find a basin of water and a towel to rub across his grimy face.

The roadhouses provided a certain degree of intimacy for the traveler, and each one had its own particular character. The innkeepers were tough, independent sorts on the whole, but each of them knew the value of a cup of coffee or a free meal for the wanderer who stumbled in wet and cold. On more than one occasion, a roadhouse operator would go out into the cold in the middle of the night to bring in a lost traveler. Alaskans depended on this kind of "bush hospitality," and they offered it selflessly. One never knew when one might need a helping hand.

The most important and respected travelers on the trails were the mail drivers. Whether they were Native, part Native, or white, they were usually the best dog drivers around, and they were experts at surviving in most any weather conditions. It was a tough job and carried huge risks, and this was reflected in their pay, which was about $150 a month, one of the highest in Alaska. They took their oath seriously and went out on the trail at times when no one else dared. They braved blizzards, rain, and bitter cold, and sometimes became the only contact between the isolated miner and the outside world. They understood the importance of a letter home to both the miner and the shopkeeper.

"To see the excitement that the mail from the Outside makes, to see the eagerness with which the men press up to the postmaster's desk for their letters, and the trembling hands as they are opened, and the filling eyes as they read, touches the heart," wrote one author as he watched the arrival of mail in 1897.

By law, mail drivers had the right of way and were always given the warmest seat at the roadhouse. They were served the best food and their dogs were given table scraps saved especially for them; sometimes the animals would be given beds of hay for the night. The dogs worked as hard as their drivers and everyone acknowledged that the mail would never get through without them.

In 1899, one driver on his route from Valdez in the south to Eagle in the Interior had tried to use horses instead of dogs, and eleven of his horses died in transit. Furthermore, just three letters made it through. Nothing could compare to the dog team, particularly when the weather was bad. The drivers often had to pay a penalty if their delivery was late, and they pushed themselves and the dogs to the limit.

"You'd have to be on time regardless of the weather or trail conditions," said Peter Curran, Jr., who had the mail route between Solomon and Golovin along the Bering Sea coast. "If I lost a day, I had to make a double run the next day. So I had to go no matter what the weather. . . . Sometimes in those storms you couldn't see half the team. You just had to trust your leader to keep going."

"There were days the poor dogs, they just hated to go," said another driver, Bill McCarty, who had a route in the Interior in the mid-1920s. "Going up river, against a headwind, cold. Oh. It really bothered them. But we had no choice. They had to go."

Roadhouse keepers and other travelers understood the extent of the pressure on the drivers and their dogs, and they often went out of their way to help. If it had snowed overnight, they would wake up early and tramp down the trail for more than ten miles so that the mail driver and his dogs would not have to labor through heavy drifts.

The drivers rarely took advantage of these privileges, and whenever they could, they would take passengers to neighboring villages or drop off gifts along the route. A mail driver might have as many as twenty-five dogs pulling two heavy freight sleds, or as few as five dogs pulling a light load. Either way, the mail was packed into heavy canvas bags tied shut with a drawstring and lashed down in the basket of the sled. Important mail such as bank drafts and company slips stayed in the driver's backpack. Sleigh bells were tied to the dogs' harnesses to announce their arrival and to warn a traveler that they were coming round the bend.

By the 1920s, mail drivers crisscrossed the entire territory. For the most part, they were a tough and humble lot, often identified by the gruesome stamps of their profession, an amputated finger or a toe lost to the cold, or a frostbitten nose or cheek. Some of them were legendary: one driver along the Yukon River route was reputed to have worn phonograph springs in his shoes after the ends of his feet were amputated. In the early 1900s, Big Ben Downing shared an 800-mile-long route that ran along the Yukon River between Dawson City in the Yukon Territory and Tanana, Alaska. On one of his runs, Downing fell through the ice and was dragged to safety by his dogs. It was minus 60 degrees and he had no matches, dry clothes, or even a hat. The only way to stay warm was to sprint behind the sled until he reached a roadhouse several miles away.

When he arrived, his clothes were frozen solid and had to be cut away. His face, hands, and legs were badly frostbitten and he hobbled across the floor. But despite his condition, Downing chose duty over recovery. Almost immediately he headed back out to his next destination, three hundred miles away.

When he arrived, his feet were so badly blistered and bleeding that the doctors wanted to amputate. But Downing, gun in hand, allowed them only a slight trim off the ends of four of his toes.

"Them feet and me are goin' together," he was reported to have said. "If I live I have use for them; if I can't have them I don't want to live."

If a driver failed to deliver his mail on time, it was a sure sign that there had been a mishap, and the lodgers at the roadhouse would go out and look for him.

William Mitchell, who laid down Alaska's first telegraph lines before becoming assistant chief of the U.S. Army Air Service, wrote about one particularly tragic experience. In his memoirs of Alaska,

Mitchell described a trip in which he had been dogsledding on the trail to Valdez and came across a mailman who appeared to be kneeling by his tent, head leaning over his hand. The mailman's lead dog, a large black Newfoundland mix, sat by his side.

"I called to the man but received no response, and going closer found that he was frozen to death. The mail was in the sled under him. Between his teeth was a match and between his knees was a box where he had tried to scratch the match when his hands had frozen."

Mitchell recalled seeing an open hole in the ice several yards behind and realized what had happened. There were pieces of harness around the mailman's camp, evidence that the four other dogs had bitten free and fled. But the lead dog had stayed behind, by his master's side, with his four paws frozen to the ground. The loyal dog was so severely frostbitten that Mitchell had no other option but to shoot him.

BY LATE in the afternoon on January 26, Governor Bone had made his decision. He had weighed the risks of the new technology against the old and now he knew what had to be done. The serum would be brought to Nome on dogsleds. But instead of sending one team to meet Leonhard Seppala midway on the trail, he would set up a relay of the best and fastest drivers in the Interior. The teams would travel night and day with no rest, no matter how bad the conditions, until they met up with Seppala at the halfway mark.

Bone sent off one message to Dan Sutherland telling him of his decision and another to Edward Wetzler, the U.S. Post Office inspector in Nenana who had maintained daily contact with the drivers.

Please engage relay dog teams to carry [antitoxin] to Tanana and thence to Ruby there to be met by team from Nome STOP Please expedite Situation reported serious STOP Territory will meet expense.

The governor dictated a separate message to Dr. Welch informing him of the decision to go with the dogs:

Inspector Wetzler instructed to hire dog teams by relay to Ruby STOP
You will please hire dog team immediately and start it to Ruby
STOP This office doing its utmost to expedite delivery.[2]

The Northern Commercial (NC) Company was the main trading
concern in Alaska, with posts in every town along the territory's
major rivers. The company had the mail delivery contract between
Fairbanks and Unalakleet and was the only operation in Nenana
capable of locating drivers in the Interior on such short notice.
Wetzler walked over to the home of Tom Parsons, the local NC
Company agent, and asked him to get the best drivers up and onto
the trail.

The call went out across the Interior by telephone and telegraph,
and the men in the Signal Corp cabins put down their coffee mugs
and set out to find the boys of the NC Company.

At the roadhouse in Minto, a tired twenty-one-year-old Athabaskan Indian named Edgar Kallands was resting after a long haul.
He had been en route to Nenana, thirty-one miles away, and now he
was being ordered to turn back to Tolovana to take his station there
and prepare for the journey to the village of Manley Hot Springs. He
had been looking forward to seeing "the big city" and taking a long
rest. But before the sweat on his gloves had dried, he was up again and
ready for the call.

Fifty-nine miles to the west, another Indian by the name of
Johnny Folger was instructed to take the serum to Tanana, the geographical center of Alaska, where the Yukon and Tanana rivers converged. From there, the message was relayed down the line to the
villages along the Yukon—Kallands, Nine Mile Cabin, Kokrines, and
Ruby—where other men were ordered to prepare. Sam Joseph, a
stocky Athabaskan, hitched up his dogs and moved out to take up his
post. Harry Pitka, a mail driver born in a spruce bow tent and raised
by a medicine man, learned of the relay as he sat watching his wife

2. The references to Ruby in Bone's telegrams are confusing: Seppala had been
asked to meet the relay in Nulato, 100 miles west of Ruby.

make a new pair of moccasins. His job would be to cover the thirty-mile leg to Ruby, and he hooked up his string of seven dogs without a moment's hesitation. Pitka was twenty-seven, and he had had a tough life. He was severely short on money, but he did not think twice about this volunteer mission.

WHILE THE mushers made hurried preparations to reach their stations, Thompson learned of Bone's decision and was furious. Marching off to his typewriter, he banged out a shrill editorial:

"Governor Bone has evidently taken charge," "Wrong Font" wrote in the January 27 issue of the *News-Miner*. ". . . Fairbanks is standing by, ready with airships and men, to cut Nome's waiting time in half if Washington wires the orders 'go. . . .' Fairbanks, only four hours away by airship . . . must sit by the fire and vision [*sic*] the Nome babies and their pioneering parents strangling and dying most horrible deaths, and no help for them. It almost makes a pioneer 'see red.' "

Thompson would have been the last person to sit idly by. In a secret vow to himself, he swore that if Fairbanks Airplane could not deliver the first batch of 300,000 units, then the company would deliver the second batch of 1.1 million units. He geared up for a protracted fight, determined not to let any official, politician, or Mother Nature stand in the way. He took aim at Bone in particular, regarding him as a traitor to the Alaskan pioneering spirit. As one acquaintance once said in a reference to Thompson's tenacity and appetite for battle: "Woe unto the public official who in his public duty was false to his trust. It were better he had not been born."

"Fairbanks could help Nome or its people would smash trying to," Thompson wrote in his paper,

> . . . if Washington could listen to Delegate Sutherland and realize that the Friendly North has passed from the dog team stage into the airship class. . . . The dog's a noble animal, man's best friend. He sticks and he'll go through with everything he has in him but along

some lines he has his limits. He will haul himself blind and misshapen for man, his master; work for nothing and steal his food, anxious to serve and loyal all the time. But it is demonstrated beyond a shadow of a doubt that in cases of great emergency the dog should be allowed to sit by the fire and dream old days over again, while gasoline and flying machines do the work that kills him.

By deciding in favor of a musher and his dogs and against an air rescue, Bone had chosen to bet against the modern age, a choice that not only went against Thompson but pitted the governor against the Zeitgeist. At a time when American innovation and ingenuity were changing the world with production lines and radio communication, Bone had put his faith in the folk wisdom of Alaska's Natives. The vast majority of mushers who would have to risk their lives were Athabaskans and Eskimos, and the rest were white men who had taken almost all their survival cues directly from the Natives.

By 1925, most Native Alaskans had made their pact with the modern age. They still hunted, fished, and traded on occasion, but their bread and butter was in hauling supplies and carting the U.S. mail along the trails. These were skills handed down to them by their parents and their grandparents.

If the serum could rescue Nome from the ravages of an ancient plague, then its safe arrival by dogsled would be a testament to the hard-learned survival skills and spirit of the Athabaskans and Eskimos.

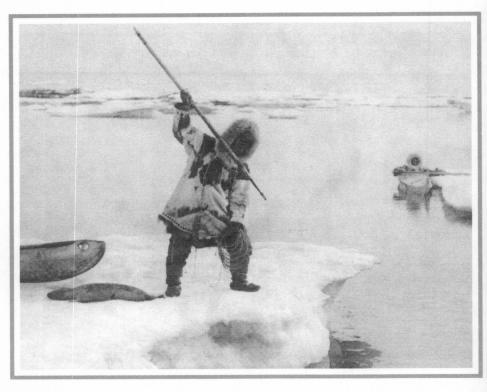

A portrait of an Eskimo hunter harpooning a seal. The ingenious adaptations of Alaska's Native inhabitants were the secret to survival in the north.

(Glenbow Archives/Lomen Collection/NC-1-48)

6

Hunters of the North

"Only those who go to the Eskimo country find that they have to submit to the discipline arctic nature enforces, and in the end they become, in some ways, like the Eskimo."
—ALASKA NATURALIST SALLY CARRIGHAR, *Moonlight at Midday*

THE DECISION to go with dogs to bring relief to Nome revealed a fundamental truth about Alaskan life: In 1925, the machine had not yet been built that could match the endurance, speed, and reliability of men and dogs. The airplane might be the way of the future, but for the people of Nome the dog team was the only hope for the present. If the epidemic was to be stopped, the rescue effort would have to rely on one of the oldest methods of transportation ever developed, along a network of footpaths and dog trails first blazed by the ancient peoples of the Arctic.

Dogsledding had evolved in the Arctic over thousands of years as an integral part of an aboriginal culture well suited to the harshest climate and living conditions on earth. Isolated and unknown to the rest of the world, both the Athasbaskan Indians of the Interior and the Eskimos along the coast learned to survive by utilizing all of the limited resources at their disposal. The land, sea, and ice provided their food, clothing, tools, and shelter. Making much out of virtually nothing, their remarkable innovations in this most unforgiving environment rank as one of the high water marks of human achievement and ingenuity.

When outsiders first arrived with the vast riches of Western technology, some naive whites were convinced they had nothing to learn from "primitive savages" barely beyond the Stone Age. Careful observers knew otherwise. In 1921, Vilhjalmur Stefansson published a best-selling account of his five-year expedition in the Arctic, *The Friendly Arctic*. His theme was a simple one: the Arctic could be as friendly and hospitable as virtually any place on earth if one only learned to adapt to local conditions and adopt local clothing and technology that had successfully evolved over thousands of years. His common-sense idea was to profit from the lessons of thousands of years of arctic evolution. This simple but profound notion is a key to the history of the modern exploration of Alaska and the Arctic: the explorers who learned Native ways of survival were most likely to survive. The reverse was equally true.

On a flat map Alaska appears to be at the end of the earth, but historically it lies at the crossroads of one of the great migration routes in world history. Most scientists believe Alaska to be the gateway through which humans came to populate America. As recently as fifteen thousand years ago, during the last Ice Age, the Bering Strait and much of the Bering and Chukchi seas were dry land, and a land bridge perhaps at least 1,000 miles wide, called Beringia, connected Siberia with Alaska. It was over this land bridge that many scientists believe the earliest subsistence hunters entered North America. These bands of "Paleo-Indians" slowly expanded across Beringia, generation by generation, hunting the large Ice Age mammals that stalked the tundra: wooly mammoths with enormous tusks, musk oxen, giant bison, moose, lions, and saber-tooth cats. Descendants of these wandering hunters eventually traversed across the entire length and breadth of the western hemisphere, reaching the tip of South America, if not even farther, as recent evidence suggests, in roughly a millennium, and are considered to be the ancestors of present-day American Indians.

Later waves of hunters included first the ancestors of the Athabaskan Indians, who today inhabit most of the boreal forest of Interior Alaska and northern Canada, and then the Eskimos, who spread across the entire Arctic as far as Greenland. These two great arctic peoples, Athabaskan hunters of the northern forest and Eskimo hunters on the treeless tundra, for generations waged the coldest of cold wars against each other, their territories separated by a no-man's-land that either side would cross only at their peril. As one early explorer reported, in one Eskimo band in northern Alaska, "every man who had slain an Indian was tattooed at the corners of the mouth as a mark of distinction."

An oft-repeated and widely believed myth is that the word "Eskimo" is a derogatory Indian term meaning "eaters of raw flesh." As a result, Canadian Inuit have since the 1970s considered it a racial slur. In fact, the word "Eskimo" was apparently originally an inoffensive reference to snowshoes, and is still widely used in Alaska.[1] Nevertheless, the language of both sides reflects the ancient rivalry. "From Hudson Bay to Alaska," wrote the anthropologist Wendell Oswalt, "the word Eskimos applied to Indians usually meant 'Lousy People.'" The forbidding Interior of Alaska belonged to the Athabaskans, where the climate is characterized by long, dark winters and short, hot summers.[2] Cutting across the great swath of boreal forest is the Yukon River, which runs 2,300 miles from its headwaters in Canada's Pacific Coast range. It meanders across Alaska, and at the Arctic Circle it shifts dramatically from northwest to southwest, ultimately spilling into the Bering Sea.

1. In Alaska, the word "Eskimo" does not have the same negative connotations that it does in Canada. For reasons of both convenience and clarity, "Eskimo" is still widely accepted in Alaska. Alaska Eskimos include both "Inuit" or Inupiat speakers, and "Yuit" or Yupik speakers. Almost two thirds of Alaska Eskimos are Yuit. The two languages are mutually unintelligible, roughly analogous it is sometimes said to English and German. The linguistic and cultural borderline between the two great Eskimo nations lies near Unalakleet, southeast of Nome, and the Seward Peninsula, with the Inuit to the north and the Yuit to the south.
2. The range of temperature in the sub-Arctic between summer and winter can differ by as much as 180 degrees. The lowest temperature ever recorded in Interior Alaska is 80 degrees below zero and temperatures in the 50- to 60-below range are not uncommon. In the brief summer, the thermometer can hit nearly 100 degrees above zero. In the winter, snowfall tends to be relatively light—in many areas the sub-Arctic is as dry as the Sahara Desert—but due to the extremely low temperatures, what falls in September will not melt until the following April or May, so the ground is usually blanketed by several feet of snow.

Athabaskans were seminomadic hunters, gatherers, and fishermen who moved from one seasonal camp to the next throughout the year in their constant search for food. The year-round subsistence cycle often included spring salmon fishing, summer berry picking, fall and winter moose and caribou hunting. Thundering herds of caribou and the elusive moose were moving targets, however, and these hunters and fishermen of the Great Northern Forest often lived precariously close to the edge of starvation. In fact, for most of the small bands, starvation was a regular part of life; the worry was not whether food shortages would come, but when. Families had to travel hundreds of miles each year in order to live off the land.

Like guerrilla warriors, the Athabaskans not only traveled far but also light. Constantly on the move, their shelters were among the simplest of any North American Indian tribe. Conical tents, or teepees, were made by sticking a circle of thin poles into the snow and covering the structure with hides of moose sewn together. Animal skins covered the floor of the tent. A circle of stones in the center of the floor was aligned with a smokehole where the poles came together. Once a fire was lit by the rubbing of sticks, it had to be tended carefully. The hot stones contained the cooking fire and radiated heat into the dwelling. When it was time to leave, the Athabaskans quenched the fire, lifted the poles, packed up their skins, and were swiftly on the move again. To break trails through the heavy snow, they wore snowshoes made from strips of rawhide stretched across birch or spruce frames. To carry their few belongings, they designed toboggans with runners that curved up like skis. These toboggans were sometimes 30 feet in length. To assist in the hunt and to carry additional supplies, families used dogs, but most could only afford to keep a few. They simply did not have enough food to feed large teams. Among the Athabaskans at that time dogs were not used for traction to pull sledges, but were instead mainly pack animals. Dogs carried packs on their backs with pouches on both sides stuffed full of supplies or meat from the hunt.

Winters in the Alaskan Interior are nearly eight months long, and the sun makes its appearance only a few hours a day, leaving few opportunities for the hunter to find anything alive. The Athabaskans, it was said, were always in a "rush to keep ahead of the darkness." Temperatures regularly fell to 50 below and snowstorms were not uncommon. Yet the snow, to an expert, was like a road map that revealed the faint movements and whereabouts of animal life. With one shot from his bow and arrow or a stone-pointed spear thrown through the heart of a moose, the hunter could feed his family through a winter. But more likely there would be few sightings of any animals in winter, and those sighted had their own adaptations to help them avoid becoming a convenient target. And so, to protect against starvation, the Athabaskans built caches on high wooden platforms and placed these strategically at different seasonal camps. Stored inside these caches were precious dried salmon and preserved moose meat.

Generation by generation, the wandering Athabaskan tribes built up a set of survival skills. They could tell you where to find every bend in hundreds of miles of river and where were the best places to catch salmon. They taught their children to test the thickness—and safety—of frozen river or lake ice by poking the point of a spear into the ice and judging the level of resistance. They created shortcuts through the Interior by using portages that served as overland connections between rivers. If you lost your way in the forest, your best chance of reorienting yourself was to climb the tallest tree in hopes of spotting and recognizing a distant outline of a particular lake or the profile of a particular mountain. Many families simply disappeared without a trace. But danger or no danger, the Athabaskans entered the forests often. For there they found one of the resources most important to their survival: stands of spruce trees.

Besides being river dwellers, residents of the boreal forest were a people of the "spruce age," using the ubiquitous evergreen trees for their shelters, bedding, caches, canoes, drying racks, tent frames, sleds, snowshoes, snares, poling sticks, weapons, and lashing, as well as chewing gum, disinfectant, and medicinal soup. The spruce tree was the all-purpose construction material and energy source of the north; its most essential purpose might have been for firewood, providing both heat and light through the eight months of winter darkness. At 50 degrees below zero, heat was even more precious for immediate survival than food or water.

In light of its unparalleled importance, the spirit of the white spruce tree possessed a special power and significance. Among the Koyukon Athabaskans, the anthropologist Richard Nelson learned, the white spruce spirit was like an omnipresent fairy godmother protecting weary travelers and warding off evil spirits. A white spruce should never be cut down for a trivial reason, as its spirit was the equal "of the most powerful animals; but it differs in having mostly benign effects on humans. . . . People can use the spirit power of white spruce trees in several beneficial ways," Nelson wrote. "The great old trees, with thick trunks and outstretched boughs, protect those who sleep beneath them."

Given their special relationship with trees, most Athabaskans were naturally fearful to be caught out in bad weather on the open tundra without a forest blanket for fuel, orientation, and shelter. For an Athabaskan, any tree was a welcome sight in a storm. Many Eskimos, on the other hand, had a much different view of life in the woods.

Just as the wandering Athabaskan tribes, who together blazed an intricate network of trails, were at home in the northern forests, the Eskimos who settled generally along the arctic coastline were equally at home along the ice-choked waters of the Bering Sea and the Arctic Ocean. Anthropological literature is filled with praise for the ingenuity and accomplishments of the Eskimos. In Wendell Oswalt's phrase, the Eskimos were "imperialists of the North," who held the distinction as "the most widely dispersed aboriginal people in the world." Richard Nelson credited them as "one of the most successful peoples in all of human history. . . . They had pushed the human animal to the northernmost limits of its endurance. They had learned to live on the sparest resources, in the virtual absence of external warmth, where the sun vanished for months on end and where no moment of life was brought without the fullest use of the human genius."

Not all Eskimos made their traditional homes in the high Arctic or on the treeless tundra; this was especially true in western Alaska, where the Eskimos often lived along coastal rivers hundreds of miles from the Bering Sea shore. However, thousands of Eskimos did permanently reside on lands in the extreme north where no other people on earth had the skill or knowledge to survive, on lands where it was too cold or too windy for any but the smallest of trees or bushes to grow.

The Eskimos actually favored an environment that most other humans would consider unbelievably harsh and desolate. Tundra-dwelling Eskimos literally preferred not to see the forest or the trees. Unlike the Athabaskans, coastal Eskimos believed the forest to be evil, and imagined the woods were alive with the sounds of tormented spirits. When the Danish explorer Knud Rasmussen made his legendary trek by dogsled across the Arctic in the 1920s, an Eskimo chief described the dangers that lurked in the trees. "It is our belief that the trees in a forest are living beings," a man named Igjugarjuk told Rasmussen, "only that they cannot speak; and for that reason we are loath to spend the night among them. And those who have at some time had to do so, say that at night, one can hear a whispering and groaning among the trees, in a language beyond our understanding."

Besides their remarkably different attitude toward trees, many aspects of Eskimo culture differed from that of the northern Athabaskans in other obvious respects. Even confused European explorers, guilty of the biggest geographical blunder in history by labeling every native group they encountered in the Americas since 1492 as "Indians," recognized from their first encounters in Greenland that the Eskimos were a people apart from all others in the New World, if only because of the environment in which they lived.

Elements of what would later come to be identified as Eskimo culture—especially the production of skin-covered kayaks and specialized harpoons to hunt marine mammals such as walrus, seal, and later whales—began to emerge on the shores of the Bering Sea about four thousand years ago. "Beyond this," the anthropologists S. A. Arotiunov and William Fitzhugh point out, "the trail of Eskimo origins vanishes in the Bering Sea fog."

What most distinguished the Eskimos from other groups was their ingenuity. Some anthropologists claim that among all of the hunting-and-gathering people on earth, the Eskimo exhibited by far the greatest technical sophistication and "technological elaboration." Near the top of any list of Eskimo innovations is the kayak. These small, lightweight skin boats were remarkable for their speed and maneuverability. Exploring Greenland in 1612, William Baffin observed that "they will row so swiftly that it is almost incredible; for no ship in the world is able to keepe way with them. . . ." A pair of Eskimo sunglasses, a wooden mask with small eye slits, protected travelers exceedingly well against snow-blindness, and "ice creepers" attached to boots let a hunter cross the slickest ice in a high wind.

The classic igloo, the dome-shaped house of snow with windows made of ice, is probably the most famous Eskimo adaptation to the arctic environment. Warmed by body heat and small stone lamps, a well-built igloo could be relatively warm and comfortable, even if the outside temperatures were 40, 50, or even 60 degrees below zero. Snowhouses came to stand to the outside world as *the* symbol of Eskimo culture. In reality, however, the vast majority of coastal Eskimos never lived in a snowhouse and never even saw one. They were common in central Canada where snow conditions were just right, but in Alaska, *iglus*—the word simply means "house"—were made of sod and the snow igloo was completely unknown. The Danish author and arctic explorer Peter Freuchen came to Alaska in 1932 with an MGM film crew to shoot the movie *Eskimo*, the first feature film ever made in the Inupiaq language. To his grave disappointment, none of the local Eskimos he found in Alaska, unlike those he knew from his years in Greenland and Canada, had ever seen an igloo, let alone knew how to build one. As a result he was forced to construct a village of igloos for the movie shoot all by himself.

Houses, or *iglus*, in Alaska were more often semisubterranean wood- or whalebone-framed dwellings covered with sod. Like today's skylights, a seal-intestine window let the light in and, when opened, served as a chimney to let smoke from the burning stone lamps escape. The dome-shaped living area was connected to a long underground tunnel entrance. Living underground was the best protection against the climate; outside cold air, trapped by the low passageway, never reached the raised living room. Seal-oil lamps, carved from soapstone into an oval shape as if to cup the palm of a hand, burned with wicks of dried moss, providing warmth and light. Food, harnesses, sleds, hunting equipment, and clothing were stored along the length of the entranceway in small compartments. These semisubterranean houses were only for winter months; come summer, when the frozen ground thawed and the houses were flooded, the Native families moved on to their annual summer fishing camps.

The Eskimos elaborated the craft of fur and skin sewing into an art, a science, and a religion. Fur and skin clothing not only enabled them to move about comfortably in the coldest of temperatures; it also served a variety of social functions as well, demarcating tribes, social standing, gender, and spiritual beliefs. Because all of their clothes came from the animals they hunted, and the success of the hunt was seen as dependent on the willingness of the prey to sacrifice themselves for the benefit of humans, the preparation, maintenance, and wearing of animal clothing took on crucial importance.

Women in the Eskimo community were the seamstresses; no job was more important for the family's survival. Without properly sewn and maintained boots, pants, and parkas, no hunter could hunt, so making the clothing for her family was the measure of a wife's worth. The work literally was never done, because the clothes had to be inspected, repaired, and maintained every day. The slightest tear while out hunting could lead to death.

Training as a skin sewer began at an early age. A young girl practiced on dolls made by her father. Once the girl married, a caring husband might carve and personalize the necessary tools to specially fit the contours of her hand, items such as ivory and bird-bone sewing needles, stone knives, caribou bone–skin scrapers, and caribou-antler snow beaters to keep the clothing dry. A healthy set of teeth was also among a woman's most important tools, as she would have to chew skins and boots to make them soft and pliable. While excavations of prehistoric graves have revealed that male skeletons show clear signs of damage akin to "tennis elbow" from overuse (probably from repeated throwing of spears and harpoons), female skeletons have been found with teeth worn down to bare stubs from years of skin chewing.

The Athabaskans had an elaborate system for preparing the skins, including rubbing them down with a paste made from decayed caribou liver or decayed brains, but the Eskimos generally achieved better results than their neighbors in the Interior with only a fraction of the time and effort. Tools used for dressing the skins typically included a stone scraper, a wood-frame skin stretcher, and a tub of urine, which was used as an all-purpose soap, shampoo, and solvent.

After the flesh and fat were scraped off, the skins were rolled in a bundle with the hairs inside, and kept in the house, as one early ethnologist said, "until they become sour and the hair loosens." The hair was then scraped off the skins and they were lashed onto a driftwood frame stretcher and placed outside to dry. Most clothing and boots had the hair left on. Typically, these skins were soaked in urine after the flesh and fat were removed, and only then went through the final scraping, stretching, and drying.

Caribou or reindeer skins made the best fur parkas, pants, and mittens because the fur is thick but the individual hairs are hollow, rendering the garment both lightweight and extremely warm. Sealskin was typically the material of choice for waterproof clothing of any type. In some areas, caribou pants were worn with the hair facing inward during cold weather, which would trap air for added insulation, and then facing outward during warmer weather. The key to the system of staying warm was to dress in layers with differing thicknesses in fur, in order to regulate the temperature next to the body, never getting too warm or too cold. Sweating was as potentially dangerous as freezing, so overheating was to be avoided at all costs. Layering also allowed moisture to be wicked away from the body, to condense on one of the outer layers, keeping the skin warm and dry. While outer garments, such as the parka, were traditionally made with the fur facing out, the inner layer of undergarments, often made from newborn or sometimes unborn fawns, was usually worn with the fur on the inside.

The parka was pulled over the head like a tunic and fitted loosely, to allow air to circulate. Stranded travelers could easily take their arms out of the sleeves and hold them against their chests to provide more warmth. A paper-thin waterproof garment made from strips of dried seal intestine was often worn over fur clothing in the winter or in wet weather during the spring. Drawstrings closed off the wrists and neck to prevent water from entering the jacket, and the bottom of the jacket covered the mouth of the kayak so that a hunter rolling in heavy seas was protected against water entering his vessel.

Eskimo fur boots, or mukluks, had caribou-fur tops and caribou-skin or waterproof sealskin soles. These were among the most durable and effective items in their clothes closet, equal or superior to any boots now manufactured. No other item of clothing was more important than a pair of boots. When confronted with dropping temperatures, the traveler could always remove his outer mittens to rub his hands and restore circulation, but boots remained on the feet at all times to keep the traveler warm and dry.

In making mukluks, the Eskimo women tried to use only one thread, with small stitches. They were careful never to make any unnecessary holes with the sewing needle. Tapering sinew thread was the key to perfectly waterproof boots. The thread was twisted so that it had a smaller diameter on one end than the other; when wet, the sinew expanded and plugged up the holes. Caribou socks or boot liners made of woven grass would absorb sweat or any additional moisture, and were taken out to dry at the end of each day.

Keeping dry was not only the secret to staying safe and comfortable on the trail; it was also essential to protect fur clothing from deteriorating. If fur clothes became damp, it wasn't as easy as hanging them by the fire to dry out, because that would make them shrink, and ill-fitting clothes could prove fatal. One trick was to beat off any snow or frost collected in the clothing before entering the heat of a house. As the inside layer wicked away the moisture from the skin, frost might likely have gathered on the inside of the outer coat, which needed to be scraped before going indoors.

. . .

THE KILLING of animals and the skinning of their flesh to provide clothes for the hunter and his family were part of an endless cycle in which death was the source of all life. Eskimos believed the natural world was alive with spirits—some kind and some malevolent—that influenced or controlled their everyday lives. Humans and animals shared a spiritual continuum that defined their universe; humans were not created to dominate the world, but to collaborate with all of the other creatures in it. In such a world, there were no hard and fast boundaries between people and animals, or even between animate and inanimate objects. Ravens and humans, salmon and seals, caribou and bears, ivory and wood, wind and rain, all possessed an equal spiritual essence, which might be transformed under the right circumstances. As a result of this ambiguous dividing line between the human and the non-human world, all creation deserved the utmost care and respect, or there would be angry spirits to pay.

The elaborate hunting traditions were in many ways ritualized offerings to animal spirits so they would continue to come to the hunter. After killing a seal, a hunter was sure to pray to its spirit and offer thanks for its sacrifice; his wife would offer its "thirsty soul" a sip of water, saying, "See, our water here is tasty, very inviting," in the fervent hope that such hospitality would encourage seals to continue coming to the village. The hunter's clothing had to be beautiful, and its stitching perfect, to please the animal spirits he was hunting. A poor seamstress with irregular stitching might drive the animals away. To further ensure a successful hunt, a seamstress never worked on clothes while her husband was out hunting, believing her inactivity would make the prey inactive.

Young women were often warned against looking a hunter in the eye so as not to deplete his power to hunt. While in bed, a wife was not to sleep facing her husband, "lest the braid of her hair appear hanging in front of his face and subsequently block his vision." Likewise, Eskimos showed respect to the wise old man in the moon who watched over the world by not looking him in the eye. Hunters often carried amulets carved out of ivory in the shape of the animals the family depended on for its survival. These charms could call the animals to the hunter, or increase the hunter's powers to hear the click-ing of caribou feet far off in the distance. The seamstress also carried charms that hung from her needlecase or caribou teeth strung from her belt that could protect her family from sickness and harm.

Animal skins empowered those wearing them with the character-istics of that animal; the hunter became part caribou, seal, wolf, or walrus by adorning himself in their clothing. With skin from a cari-bou's legs on his boots, he was sure to emulate the speed of a running caribou, while a wolf or wolverine belt with the tail hanging down his back would give him their strength and courage as a hunter. A wooden hunting hat with baleen enabled a kayaker "to pass safely through the currents like a whale," while the wood from the land ensured he would return safely again to solid ground.

Emulating the manners and habits of wild animals had a practical as well as a spiritual side, because successful hunters were those who knew best what they were hunting for. The various species of seal—particularly the Ringed and Bearded Seals—were perhaps the most widespread and useful animals in the entire Eskimo world. In addi-tion to being a reliable and widely available food source for both men and dogs, these ubiquitous marine mammals supplied Eskimos with skins for boots and kayaks, and oil for heating, lighting, and cooking. Seal meat, seal oil, seal blubber, and sealskin could supply most of a family's needs for food, fuel, clothing, and shelter.

The Eskimo hunted seals with a variety of different methods both on the ice and in the water. One traditional technique was to stalk a sleeping seal as it napped on the ice pack, requiring the hunter to approach within harpoon distance—about 15 feet—of his prey. As the seals were not afraid of other seals, the hunter crawled forward pre-tending to be a seal himself, sliding and scratching, moving his arms like flippers and his head like an anxious seal scouting for polar bears, as he moved in for the kill.

Living off the land, the ice, and the sea, a man naturally grew expert at reading and studying animal behavior, as well as terrain, ice conditions, and weather patterns. Though it is not true, as a well-known myth claims, that the Eskimo language has an extraordinary number of words for snow, it is true that the Natives did have a remarkably detailed and specific knowledge of snow and ice conditions. This was essential for their day-to-day survival, because the arctic environment poses innumerable hazards, and too often the smallest mistake in judgment could mean death. In a land with no readily available shelter and no easily distinguishable landmarks—the flatness of the arctic coastal plain makes Kansas look like Switzerland—it was remarkably easy to get lost or disoriented. Sometimes the only way a lost traveler could tell what direction he was going was to feel the contours of snowdrifts in the dark, trying to find the patterns left by the prevailing winds. An experienced traveler knew which way the winds blew, and used them not only to predict future weather but to serve as a beacon to bring him home.

The hardest going of all was across the ice. No camp on the floating ice was ever completely safe, no matter how stable it appeared. Driven by winds and currents the moving ice is a churning, shape-shifting platform, in a constant state of flux, expanding and contracting with the seasons. The top of the world is covered every winter by nearly 7 million square miles of ice, an area about twice the size of the entire United States, of which close to 2 million square miles is destroyed each summer, to grow back again the following winter. The constant cycle of fragmenting and congealing at the mercy of the winds leaves behind long cracks, pressure ridges, and piles of icy rubble. The World War II Army Air Corps *Arctic Manual* warns that the surface of the ice resembles "something between a system of miniature mountain ranges and the interior of a granite quarry."

Whether on land or ice, the power and fury of an arctic winter storm, like a biblical plague, dwarfs all human capacity to withstand it. Extremely cold temperatures may be unpleasant, yet the greatest arctic hazard is not the cold but the wind speed. Wind is the great dictator of northern life. On the trail, almost nothing protects a man from the wind, and in the face of an arctic gale it is easy to understand why some Natives believed the wind to be a malevolent spirit. A trail-hardened pioneer missionary would later claim that he could travel with relative comfort at 65 degrees below zero in calm air, but he always feared and detested the winds on the Bering Sea coast. "One grows to hate that wind," he wrote, "with something like a personal animosity, so brutal, so malicious does it seem."

Patience was the greatest virtue for the arctic traveler, because the only way to beat the wind was to wait it out. Sometimes the best step to take was simply to sit down and go to sleep. Vilhjalmur Stefansson told the story of an old Eskimo woman caught out in a sudden storm only half a mile from her home. The blowing snow enveloped her and in a matter of seconds she could not see further than a few feet in any direction. Instead of panicking and exhausting herself in a fruitless search for her house, she remained calm and sat down in the lee of an ice hummock to get out of the raging wind. Sitting on her fur gloves to keep her seat warm, she took her arms out of her sleeves and crossed them against her chest, leaning forward to reduce her surface space, much the way dogs instinctively curl up into a tight ball, and she soon went to sleep. Whenever she got too chilled, she awoke and jumped up to restore her circulation, before crouching down again behind the ice hummock. For more than seventy hours she kept sitting, jumping, stretching, and sleeping, before the storm finally abated, and she could clearly see her home only a few minutes away. The lesson according to Stefansson was simple. If you get lost in a blizzard, the old Eskimo way offers the best chance of survival: Keep calm, keep still, keep dry, and keep sleeping until the weather clears.

OF ALL the great Eskimo innovations in hunting and traveling, probably none was more important than their use of dogs. Dogs became the Eskimos' "sixth sense," their extra nose, ears, and eyes, which could smell a seal or hear a caribou long before a mere human. The dog made life possible for the Eskimos in the Arctic. "Without dogs," as the ethnologist E. W. Nelson wrote in 1887, "the larger portion of the great Eskimo family peopling the barren northern coast of America would find it impossible to exist in its chosen home."

When the first dog walked across the Bering Land Bridge more than ten thousand years ago, he did not come alone. Dogs and humans arrived in Alaska together, and into modern times the partnership between them has been one of the keys to survival in the north. Around the world dogs have served as hunters, sentries, and companions since before the dawn of recorded history; but no one ever learned to harness the power of dogs as effectively as the Eskimos did. The greatest technological leap came in relatively recent times, when the Eskimos put dogs together with sleds and perfected the art of dog traction. "The dog team," as one expert claimed, "is one of the most effective devices ever invented by man." Like the horse on the Great Plains and the camel in the desert, the dog was the cornerstone of the Eskimo way of life in the arctic ice and snow.

Dogs are the oldest domesticated animals on earth, though no one really knows how many tens of thousands of years *Canis familiaris* has been man's best friend. It was probably during the Paleolithic Age that tamed wolves began gradually to evolve into dogs, and humans have been living with these "wolves in dogs' clothing" ever since.[3] The man-dog contract goes back to before the invention of writing, before the invention of the wheel, even before the invention of agriculture. In that sense, living with dogs may be one of the oldest surviving cultural landmarks of our heritage, a surviving fragment of the Stone Age.

Many Native American tribal myths depicted humans as descendants of wolves or dogs. One myth from the lower Yukon held that the mother of all humans was a she-wolf who married a man. "In the beginning there was water over all the earth," the legend runs, "and it was very cold; the water was covered with ice, and there were no people." Into this frozen land came a man "from the far side of the great water," who took the wolf for his wife in the hills along the Bering Sea coast north of the Yukon River, and they had many sets of twins, each

---

3. The relationship between prehistoric man and wolves, as explored in Mark Deer's *Dog's Best Friend: Annals of the Dog-Human Relationship* (New York: Henry Holt, 1997), dates back thousands of years to when nomadic hunters selectively bred wolves who possessed characteristics favorable for helping them in bringing down large mammals.

with one male and one female, who spoke different languages. "The twins peopled the earth with their children. . . . "

Other ancient legends from Native Alaska date the alliance between man and dog back to the creation of the earth. When the world was being formed, one story goes, the earth split in half and a great chasm separated all of the earth's animals on one side and man on the other. All of the beasts took flight except for one animal: the dog. Standing at the edge of the abyss, the dog began to bark and howl and plead to the other side until the man shouted, "Come!" When the dog had hurled himself across the chasm to reach the other side, he clung to the "far edge" before man pulled him up by his two front paws. "Had it not been for man, the dog would certainly have been lost forever."

Whether it was the dogs that owed their existence to humans, or the other way around, the collaboration between Eskimos and dogs certainly kept both alive through many thousands of long cold winters. Some archeologists believe that initially dogs were predominately kept as a walking larder to provide meat and fur for traveling Eskimo tribes. A Russian explorer along the Bering Sea coast in the 1830s claimed that two delicacies in high demand among the Natives were "fermented fish-heads of salmon . . . and fattened young dog." Besides supplying fur and a diet of meat, the Eskimos also used dogs for hunting, navigating, and packing supplies.

As hunting dogs, they were invaluable in tracking bears or finding tiny breathing holes for seals on the pack ice. When the pack ice thickened enough that the seals could no longer break through its thin surface with the top of their heads, they gnawed at the thickening ice with their teeth, tunneling holes that were up to seven feet in depth, but on the surface just big enough to stick their nostrils up against the hole to breathe. These breathing holes might have been invisible to the naked eye, but not to the dogs' keen sense of smell. Hunters from a village would span out on foot in every direction across the frozen ice with their sealing dogs, whose heads hung low to sniff out snowdrifts and ridges along the surface of the ice as the animals led the hunters on a zigzag course. The hunter walked behind his dog for a mile or more out from shore, then the dog would suddenly stop. The hunter poked through the soft drift of snow with his ivory rod until he indeed felt it dip into the hole hidden below. Next, the hunter would position himself on the downwind side of the hole. There he would wait, sometimes for hours, for the seal to rise near the surface, and then quickly spear it when the seal inevitably came up through the ice for air. The dog waited all the while beside his hunter, knowing from experience that his job was not yet done.

Hunters from the village might come over to help pull out the seal if it was too much struggle for one man to haul out his 800-pound load. After hauling his prey from the water, the hunter would hitch the dead seal by a leather trace to the leather harness on his trusted dog, who would drag it a mile or two back to camp by himself while the hunter went across the ice to where a neighboring hunter stood over another seal hole. "The dog does this errand with the greatest of goodwill," one early explorer wrote, "for he knows that he is going to get a feed at the end of it."

Though no one really knows when or where Eskimos first began hitching dogs to sleds, the scant evidence indicates that they copied the practice from Siberian Natives, perhaps as much as a thousand or five hundred years ago. Over the generations they developed various lightweight sleds, harnesses, and other equipment, using materials such as driftwood, rawhide, walrus tusk, caribou antlers, and whalebone. Early explorers recorded the ingenuity of seal-skin socks that the Eskimos designed to protect the dogs' feet and legs against rough ice. Some sledges even had runners coated with ice. It was a laborious process to make ice shoes for a sledge, and the ice had to be reapplied frequently because travel wore it away; but the result was far superior at the time to any other available material. To prepare the surface, the traveler smeared the wood skis on which the sled would run with an icy paste made from peat or moss mixed with water. Once this was frozen, he applied a final coat of warm water that quickly froze to form the ice runners that would glide across the snow.

Initially, most Eskimos families usually had few dogs; three or fewer was common because they did not have the food to feed them.

Ordinarily, the dogs were quite territorial, but they were seldom if ever tied up, so that they could forage for their own meals on rodents, squirrels, and feces. With such small teams most travelers never rode on the sled; they were either out front with the dogs pulling or behind the sled pushing. When Lieutenant George Stoney explored the area north of the Seward Peninsula in the mid-1880s, he came upon a large Eskimo party of forty people, with fifty dogs and twelve sleds, and was astonished to see that the men, women, and dogs were all hitched together. A one-dog family in particular caught his attention. "A woman with a child on her back and a single dog with three or four puppies playing beside it would drag a sled," Stoney wrote, "while the man behind pushed and guided, yelling at the single dog as lustily as though his team comprised a dozen or more."

Relying on a combination of human power and dog power, only the bare essentials, supplies, and survival gear could be loaded on the sled. Everything had to be trimmed exactly to size. Seal meat, for instance, was butchered to fit the width of the sled for easy loading. With so few dogs, the sleds could neither haul heavy loads—on a good trail a single dog could pull at most about 75 to 100 pounds— nor travel too far. As a result, Eskimo settlements scattered along the Bering Sea tended to be small, widely dispersed, and mobile, with the people constantly following the food supply in a seasonal cycle.

For the Eskimos as well as the Indians in Alaska, the familiar cycle of life was radically altered on a July day in 1741 when Vitus Bering, a Danish sailor on a Russian ship, sighted the Alaskan mainland. It was the beginning of a tidal wave of change that would touch every aspect of Native life. Western technology, Western values, strange diseases, new religions, and alcohol all would challenge every assumption of the old ways, leaving many to believe that traditional knowledge no longer had any relevance.

People armed with clearly superior technology tend to believe they are themselves superior. A man with an iron tool is unlikely to be impressed by a man with only a stone. This was a prejudice shared by many early European explorers, who steadfastly refused to consider eating native foods or wearing aboriginal clothing, in the belief that "going native" signified a character defect and a lack of civilization. As a result, many adventurers from southern climates who eschewed fresh seal blubber for tinned beef or preferred wool coats and leather boots to fur parkas and sealskin mukluks suffered the consequences. A diet rich in raw meat provided Eskimos with a needed source of vitamin C and was further supplemented in the summers by eating berries and cooking a broth from tree bark that protected them against illness. In the absence of this diet, debilitating cases of scurvy, not to mention frostbite and lead poisoning from the solder used in canning, were inevitable pitfalls for the unprepared explorer, as shown most dramatically by the death of Sir John Franklin and the 128 men in his crew on his last expedition in 1847.

Less rigid than the military men or professional explorers were fur trappers and traders, who, because they lived among the Natives for years, were often better students of what it took to survive in the north, and less blinded by standards of "appropriate" behavior. In the late eighteenth and nineteenth centuries, Alaska was the front line where two colossal fur-trading empires collided: the Russians from the west, and the British Hudson's Bay Company across Canada from the east. Though the fur traders were relatively few in number, the wealth of trade goods that they brought with them had an enormous impact, even on peoples hundreds of miles away with whom they never came into direct contact.

Among the many trade goods that they introduced, no single item was more important than the rifle. The introduction of firearms to a hunting society had profound implications. Most of all it meant that a man's killing power and range were vastly increased, but at a steep price. Native groups had always traded with neighboring tribes, but in general the local environment had provided the necessities of life. Now those necessities included firearms, manufactured cloth, steel needles, and cast-iron pots. What hunter would want a spear if given the chance to use a gun? To acquire the ammunition he suddenly needed, the hunter would now have to become a professional trapper, securing skins not for his family's clothing but to sell to the trader. The trading post thus often became a permanent population center and the nucleus of a future village.

Firearms and fur-trading capitalism revolutionized the use of dogs in the north, the proof of which is still evident every time a dog musher says "mush." French Canadian fur trappers in the service of the Hudson's Bay Company recognized how useful the dog traction of the Eskimos would be on a trapline. They hooked up their dog teams to toboggans and sleds, and commanded them to go in French, shouting, *"Marche!"* or *"Marchons!"* which was gradually corrupted to "Mush!" The trappers taught the Athabaskans to mush dogs and the Indians readily adopted dog traction as a superior method of moving faster and farther about the forest. Previously the Athabaskans only had small "pack" dogs, not sled dogs. But packing with a single dog was not nearly as efficient as sledding with a team of dogs; the new weapons and new demands of trading made the vast leap from packing to sledding inevitable. The new cycle had an irresistible logic. Hunger for trade goods, combined with the desire to kill more game in order to trap more furs to get more trade goods, made the adoption of Eskimo dog sledding by the Athabaskan Indians a natural development.

Among the Eskimos too the introduction of firearms and the resultant increase in hunting power and hunting range had permanent effects, including a substantial rise in dog power, which in turn facilitated the growth of larger and more permanent settlements. Armed with rifles and steel implements the Eskimos could hunt more game and catch more fish, enabling them to feed bigger and better dog teams. It was also about this time that Eskimos began to adopt the Siberian practice of using specially designated lead dogs, improving harnesses, and developing the tandem hitch. In aboriginal times in Alaska, the few dogs were usually hitched to sleds like fingers on a hand, with each dog attached to a trace directly from the sled. This "fan hitch," which is still common today in eastern Canada and Greenland, was preferred when hunting on the ice pack, but the tandem hitch was superior on land. It not only kept the dogs separate but also delivered more concentrated power to the front of the sled, and it became the universal practice in Alaska.

The increased mobility brought by the dog teams led to the concentration of population into fewer settlements, as hunters could regularly commute between various hunting and fishing grounds from a single location. A man with eight dogs could haul four times as much seal meat or travel four times as far as a man with only two. The added mobility made it more practical for the meat to be carried back to the family, instead of carrying the family to the meat.

AS FAR-REACHING as the changes wrought by the fur trade were, the handful of solitary traders in the Interior was merely the first act in a larger drama that began when outsiders learned there was gold in Alaska and the Yukon basin of Canada. Following the Klondike strike of 1896, tens of thousands of men from around the world swarmed across the ancestral lands of the Eskimos and Athabaskans, tearing up the creeks digging for gold. Ironically, it was dogs and dog traction, for centuries the mainstay of Eskimo survival, that made this new world run. During the gold rushes, dogs brought the modern world to Alaska, hauling food, mining supplies, medicine, passengers, and gold across the network of rivers and trails that Eskimos and Athabaskans had been following for hundreds of years.

In addition to trade goods, the gold rush brought some strange ideas to Alaska, and the most bizarre may have been the belief of some U.S. government officials that Alaskans would be better off living in Alaska without dogs. Ambitious entrepreneurs tried many alternative forms of transportation and communication that they hoped would be superior to dogs, including horses, goats, hot-air balloons, bicycles, ice skates, ice boats, ice trains, and passenger pigeons. But the favorite choice of several key officials was the reindeer. The man behind the reindeer project was a Presbyterian missionary, Sheldon Jackson, the head of the U.S. government's education program for Alaska, who founded the first schools among the Inupiaq Eskimo along the Bering Sea and the Arctic Ocean in 1890. Jackson feared that the depredations of the Yankee whaling fleet, which by that time had been cruising in the Bering Sea for almost half a century, had helped to decimate the marine mammals and the caribou upon which the Eskimo depended, leaving them with the prospect of imminent starvation. Meanwhile, on the Siberian side of the Bering Sea, he saw that the prosperous Native reindeer herders had plenty of stock to see them through the harshest winter. Reindeer and caribou are the same species, only reindeer are domesticated and the caribou are not. Jackson reasoned that the solution would be to "stock" the Alaskan side with Siberian reindeer that would thrive by grazing on the tundra moss, and to transform the Eskimos from caribou hunters into reindeer herders.

Alaska governor John Brady agreed with Jackson's plan wholeheartedly, and claimed that reindeer could provide "an abundance of wholesome food . . . at comparatively small effort." He believed the introduction of reindeer to Alaska was providential. "The camel," he wrote, "is no more divinely fitted for the burning desert than is [the reindeer] for the frozen north."

Beginning with the initial shipment of 171 deer in 1892, by the end of the decade with further shipments and births the total had climbed to nearly three thousand animals. Dr. Jackson was a tireless promoter of the reindeer project; in 1903 he went before Congress to argue that reindeer should replace dogs as the primary beasts of burden in Alaska, and that they even be given the responsibility of hauling the U.S. mail. In general, Jackson had a low opinion of Native culture; he believed for instance that Native languages were decadent and encouraged the policy of punishing children for speaking them. But he reserved special scorn for dogs, testifying to Congress that dogs were unreliable, treacherous beasts that "require considerable food for their support, while reindeer are gentle, timid and eat little, foraging on the moss and spruce of the tundra."

Dr. Jackson issued instructions for missionaries and reindeer handlers to approach these reindeer with extreme caution. While harnessing the reindeer, Jackson warned, it is best not to touch them if you can avoid it. Simply hurl the harness over their neck from as far a distance as possible and then pull the rope back as if tightening a noose. One obedient missionary found the reindeer were reluctant to follow any orders. "With many misgivings I finally perched myself on top of the loaded sled behind the reindeer, which I was to drive," he wrote. "At first there was no trouble, but as soon as I attempted to guide the deer, my efforts were treated with contempt. No matter how hard nor how often I pulled on the line he paid no attention to it, except by occasionally coming to a full stop and turning around to look at me in a manner that made me feel rather uncomfortable, for the front hoofs of the deer are formidable weapons."

Among the many people who decried Dr. Jackson's campaign against Alaskan sled dogs was Archdeacon Hudson Stuck, a missionary who believed that the Natives did not have to be remade in the image of white men. He preached that the Native languages, cultures, and traditions were worthy of honor and respect, and that no dog is a "savage beast . . . unless he happens to belong to a savage beast." Upon Dr. Jackson's urging, the government did try to deliver the mail on some Alaskan routes with reindeer, and a "deluded prospector" or two tried to use reindeer instead of dogs, but Stuck claimed it did not take long to see the absurdity of the plan. The reindeer "were soon abandoned on the mail trails, and the prospector, after one season's experience, slaughtered his reindeer and traded its meat and hide for a couple of dogs."

Writing in 1914, Hudson Stuck believed that it would be rash to predict that the dog team would ever be completely abandoned on the trails of Alaska. He thought that so long as the salmon swims and the prospector lives, so long as the Indians move about the great arctic wilderness, and so long as "quick travel over great stretches of country is necessary," then "so long will the dog be hitched to his sled in Alaska."

Eleven years later, the decision to go with the dogs to rush the serum to Nome would prove that Hudson Stuck was right.

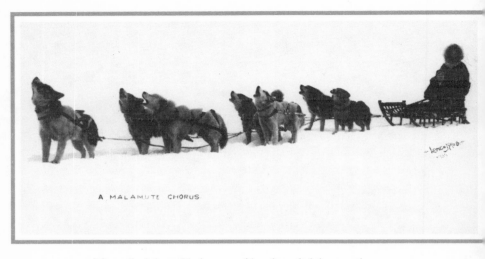

A MALAMUTE CHORUS.

The call of the wild. A team of howling sled dogs ready to run.
(Anchorage Museum of History and Art/B72.88.44)

7

The "Rule of the 40s"

"It takes a Northman to survive the North. Not only the cold . . . but the terrible, silent menace of it, the soundless days without end, when the thought of being the only human in some vast stretch of its white wastes is too terrifying a thought for one companion-loving human to carry, and keep his mental balance."

— BERT HANSEN, A U.S. DEPUTY MARSHAL
OF ALASKA'S INTERIOR

SIX HUNDRED and seventy-four miles east of Nome, "Wild Bill" Shannon waited impatiently inside the two-room railroad station at the Interior town of Nenana. It was Tuesday, January 27, just shy of 9:00 P.M., and he had been awaiting the serum from Dr. Beeson in Anchorage. The locomotive had left Anchorage with the 20-pound package almost twenty-four hours ago and it was due to arrive at any moment.[1]

1. Running a railroad in the Alaskan Interior was no easy endeavor. Blizzards often blocked the tracks, and the cold temperatures created frost heaves and an icy coat over the equipment. The old locomotives, built in 1906, were originally intended for Panama, so the engine car where coal was shoveled into the firebox was open and unprotected from the elements. "These storms are of such severity that they have often blown the windows out of the engine cabs and sent our men to hospitals for months with pneumonia," a railroader told reporters in January 1925. "Many times engine men have been lifted bodily from their open cabs, being so overcome with cold as to be incapable of moving" (*Anchorage Daily Alaskan*, January 31, 1925).

Nenana was the second to last town on the 470-mile-long railroad, which started at the southern port of Seward on a bay off the Gulf of Alaska and ended in Fairbanks. Long ago Nenana had been an Athabaskan Indian settlement at the confluence of two major Interior waterways, the Nenana and Tanana rivers, and a traditional gathering place for Indians to trade and hold their celebrations, or potlatches.[2] Over time, Nenana had its share of fur trappers, traders, and miners coming through, but it was the construction of the railroad, begun in 1915, that changed everything. By the time the railroad was completed in 1923, Nenana had become a major distribution point for goods and passengers between Alaska's southern regions and the Interior.

Nenana had been picked for the start of the serum run because it was at the junction where the railroad met the mail trail to Nome. The serum's 300-mile journey by train from Anchorage would shorten the trip by days, but once the serum arrived in Nenana, it would still have to travel the 674 miles west to Nome, clear across the territory, and there was only one way to traverse this part of Alaska in winter: by dogsled.

Lanky and fair-haired, Wild Bill was a jack-of-all-trades and, like so many other men in the territory, master of quite a few of them. He was a mail driver, miner, trapper, and fearless dog driver, who was known to have the fastest dog team in the area. His skills as a driver, combined with a combustible mixture of hot temper, sharp wit, and willingness to take risks on the trail, no doubt accounted for his nickname. Not coincidentally, he had also become a scholar of the deep freeze. Tonight, his hard-acquired knowledge and skills would be tested, perhaps as never before.

On his way to the railroad station, Shannon had sensed that the temperature was dropping well below the minus 30- to 40-degree mark that was typical for that time of year. When it was this cold, your breath formed into ice crystals and the air pinched your nostrils as you drew it in. It was like the sting of a bee, and the pain cut short

2. Some sources say that the word *Nenana* means "a good place to camp between the rivers" in the Athabaskan language.

every deep breath. Even inside the railroad station he stayed bundled up, his bearskin parka down nearly to his knees.

Had the decision been left to Edward Wetzler, the governor's man in charge of overseeing the relay, Shannon would not have set off until daybreak. By then the sunlight would have warmed the trail slightly and given the driver a clear view of it. Even so, Shannon would still be violating a rule of survival that many mushers were reluctant to challenge, but often did. Wild Bill Shannon was about to break the "rule of the 40s." The rule warned against running a dog team in temperatures below minus 40 degrees and above 40 degrees. At 40 degrees and over, a husky can get overheated and suffer from dehydration.[3] At 40 below, 2 degrees below the point at which mercury freezes, there is little room for error. Even the U.S. Army stationed in the Interior village of Tanana had forbidden its soldiers from going out on patrol when the temperature dropped so low.[4]

Tonight, it was 50 below zero.

"Traveling at 50 below is all right as long as it's *all right*" was a proverb known to many Alaskans. At this temperature, Alaska was a different world, a land with its own peculiar physics. A cup of boiling water flung into the air, for example, would become, as if by magic, a ghostly cloud of vapor. Steam rose from every finger on a bared hand as the vapor that passes continually through the pores became more visible. Spit froze, and opening the door to a warm cabin was an invi-

---

3. Panting is one way a dog can try to cool down. The hotter a dog gets, the more heavily it will pant. Panting circulates air over the mouth and tongue, which are moist, and allows for evaporation and thus heat loss. But without a sufficient amount of water, panting will work for only so long and a dog can dehydrate and overheat.

4. In the mid-1920s, Alaskans most commonly used alcohol-filled thermometers, which were often handmade and unreliable. During the Klondike gold rush, one popular pioneer trader named Jack McQuesten set outside his popular trading post four bottles, placed in the order in which they froze: quicksilver, whiskey, kerosene, and Perry Davis Pain Killer. Pioneers said that when the Perry Davis Pain Killer froze, it indicated a minimum of minus 75 degrees. Instructions for the painkiller were said to warn a traveler not to move away from the fire when the product had frozen.

tation to the phantoms. As the cold air rushed inside, moisture on the walls and floors would form into a chain of ice crystals, like tiny chandeliers in a woodshed. Outside, where the super-cooled air sucked out any lingering moisture, the landscape took on a fragile, glasslike quality. Objects would come into sharp focus and the landscape would fill with the fine, glittering crystals of hoarfrost.

In any weather condition, mushing was a dangerous profession and a driver could torture himself just thinking of ways he might die on the trail. A sweeper, or low-hanging branch, might knock out an unsuspecting driver. A moose might suddenly appear around a bend and, startled by the onrush of dogs, charge in and kill. A driver could fall and be stranded without food or supplies. He could get wet, soak his matches, and not be able to build a fire in time before the deadly freeze set in. Death waited on every stretch of river and every dip in the trail, but at minus 40 and minus 50 degrees, the chances of losing one's life increased substantially.

Stories traveled from town to town of those who had defied the cold, reminders to all who ventured out on the trail how quickly one could lose a hand or a foot. At 50 below, one driver explained, "a lost glove means a lost hand." Within minutes, an exposed hand or cheek could freeze, and a numbing toe could turn into the texture of wood. Life on the trail became a mental game against fear, a struggle between one's skill at managing the elements and the fierce determination of nature to have its way with you. Survival required a relentless vigilance, fueled by a stubborn refusal to stop fighting. To give in to weariness, to give up, meant almost certain death.

A few years earlier, along the very same trail Shannon was about to take, a trapper named Meyers had accidentally gotten his feet wet, and he had nearly paid with his life. It had been 50 below and Meyers was within a mile and a half of the telegraph station in the small settlement of Minto when he suddenly fell through the ice. Within seconds, his feet began to freeze. Soon he started to shiver uncontrollably and could not strike a match to light a fire. He ran down the trail, hoping he could somehow make it to Minto, but his pace grew slower and more erratic. He lost feeling in both feet and began to stumble over every small obstacle. He dragged himself up each time he fell, until he finally reached the telegraph station. Inside the cabin, the operator could hear the door open behind him and then "a sound as of someone pounding . . . two by fours down violently on the floor." He suddenly thought, "only one thing can make a man's feet sound like that—to be frozen solid."

Meyers survived the ordeal, but only barely—he lost both feet.

Now Shannon would be making a much longer run, half of it along the same trail that nearly killed Meyers. Ahead of him lay fifty-two miles of rough terrain over a frozen river and along steep banks to the roadhouse in Tolovana, where another dog driver would be waiting. Normally, the Nenana-Tolovana run took two days, with an overnight stop at Johnny Campbell's roadhouse in Minto. Shannon was told to cover the route in a single spurt. This would have been a challenge for any musher at any time, but in Shannon's case it was especially dangerous, because he would be working with a team of relatively inexperienced dogs.

The leader in Shannon's nine-dog crew was Blackie, a five-year-old husky with a white cross on his chest. Shannon once boasted that Blackie was the grandson of a timber wolf, which suggested a romantic combination of the wild and the tamed, with both elements working in perfect alliance. Jack London himself described such a breed, but the very notion was impractical. Wolves hunted; they did not pull. A few miners may once have succeeded in breeding a sled dog to a wolf in an attempt to produce an heir with tougher pads, more speed, and a keener sense of trail. But the wolf-dog crosses would not have been much use. Although there may have been a team or two in Alaska composed of wolf dogs, most experts agree that such hybrids were a myth. Wolf dogs tend to be intractable, aggressive, and territorial, and would have posed a danger in a team.[5]

5. The aggressiveness in wolf dogs does not necessarily come from the wolf heritage. In his book *The Company of Wolves* (New York: Alfred A. Knopf, 1995), Peter Steinhart writes that wolves tend to back off from fights and retreat from

Shannon had adopted Blackie after leaving the army, where he had served time as a blacksmith in the Alaskan Interior. Over the past few years, the dog had helped him deliver the mail, carry goods and sup-plies to his copper claims, and run the traplines in the nearby woods. By now, Shannon knew the dog's quirks, strengths, and weaknesses as well as the animal knew Shannon's.

But the eight other members of the team, all two-year-olds, were a different story. They would need close monitoring. There was Solly, a Siberian Husky with ice-blue eyes; Jimmy, the grandson of Blackie; also Princess, Cub, Jack, Jet, Bear, and Bob. They were all good, strong dogs and Shannon had raised and trained them, but they were young and relatively inexperienced. This was their first twelve-hour run in such cold temperatures, and Shannon knew the animals could become a danger to him as well as to themselves.

It would have been wiser for Shannon to wait at least until morn-ing, as Wetzler had argued, especially given the falling temperatures. But in these parts, a man did not carry the name "Wild Bill" without having earned it, and he was prepared to risk all. Across the river from the Nenana railroad station, on the steep riverbank, stood the white crosses of forty-six Athabaskan Indians who had died here during the influenza pandemic seven years earlier, a quiet reminder of how vul-nerable Native Alaskans were to the white man's diseases.

---

danger. Wolves will rarely bite a pack member. A pack would not survive con-stant aggression and therefore conflicts are usually resolved before they reach that stage.

The myth of wolf sled dog teams continued into the 1900s in Alaska and was perhaps perpetuated by breeders and drivers trying to sell their sled dogs for top prices, particularly to beginners in awe of the idea. Wolves, however, are not stronger than sled dogs, nor do they have greater endurance. The biologist and sled dog enthusiast Raymond Coppinger writes in *Dogs: A Startling New Under-standing of Canine Origin, Behavior and Evolution* (New York & London: Scribner, 2001) that breeding a sled dog to a wolf "would be at least an evolutionary digression, if not a degradation in the behaviors of both. Wolves have not been selected to be sled dogs." Contrary to popular myth, a sled dog team does not run like a pack of wolves. "A pack," writes Coppinger, "is about chasing some-thing. Sled dogs are running because other dogs are running." It is the sole

"Hell, Wetz," Shannon had told the Post Office inspector. "If people are dying . . . let's get started."

Shannon would pick up the serum as soon as it arrived and cover his share of the run tonight, no matter how cold. By early the next morning, he would either be fifty-two miles further west in the safety of the Tolovana roadhouse, or in serious trouble.

The distant chugging of the steam locomotive could be heard well before Shannon and the dogs saw the train. In this temperature, every sound reverberated through a tunnel formed between the warm air above and the heavier cold air below, traveling twice as far. Although Shannon could not see anything, the train sounded as if it were just around the corner. When it emerged from the darkness, steam gusted from the locomotive. A small crowd had gathered on the platform, among them Shannon's wife, Anna, who had come to see him off. She was a tough pioneer woman with deep blue eyes and brown hair, and she had often in the past accompanied him in his travels.

The crowd's excitement was infectious, and the dogs strained and leapt in their padded leather harnesses, tugging at the sled. Even before the train came to a complete stop, conductor Frank Knight jumped onto the platform with the 20-pound package of serum and ran over to Shannon.

---

motivation. "There is a rhythm to their run and they can hear that rhythm and they run to it," Coppinger adds. "When you stand on the back of a sled, you can feel it. It is powerful."

Coppinger discusses one zoologist and wolf expert who as an experiment tried to train hand-raised, nearly one-year-old wolves to pull a sled. Despite months of training, the wolves would not fully accept being harnessed together in such close quarters. They became territorial and when they got tired they simply lay down. They refused to take directional commands. And finally, when a robin landed among the wolves while at rest, they began to climb over each other, entangled their chains, and fought. The experiment was a failure. The zoologist ended up pulling the sled home. Basically, wolves are not suited to run in a team. Being independent-minded, they ran at their own gait and were more concerned about defending their personal space than moving forward. These traits would compromise the effectiveness of the team and the safety of the driver.

Shannon took the precious cargo and tied it down in his sled. He double- and triple-checked the harnesses and lines and made certain that the emergency supplies were all in order. Any musher worth his salt carried certain bare necessities: an ax, a blanket, a knife, rations, a tarpaulin for setting up camp, and tools for making a fire. In one pocket, he would have a waterproof container with matches, and in the other, wood shavings and dried twigs or a piece of camphor.

Satisfied that everything was in order, Shannon mounted the runners, released the sled, and took off, bolting along the tracks, down the bank to the Tanana River and into the cold, dark Interior. He had never had such a large audience watch him start a run, but tonight there was no time to think about anything but the job ahead.

High above the endless spires of spruce and birch, the stars shone with cold brilliance and the moon was a sliver in the sky, less than a quarter full.

THE ROUTE would follow the Tanana River northward in three long meandering curves for the thirty miles to Minto, an Athabaskan village in the lowlands, and then curve sharply to the west to Tolovana. It was a varied terrain of smooth surfaces and upended pieces of ice that could bruise the knees and break elbows, and the trail often required heavy pushing and frustrating lurches.

As they crossed the Tanana to the trail on the east bank, the dogs surged forward in their collars, panting heavily and leaving behind wisps of steam that hung for a moment like ghosts along the trail. On any other occasion, the veils would have been beautiful to watch, but on that evening they were a sign that the dogs were moving too fast in the severe cold. In addition, the route was in atrocious shape. A few days earlier, a horse team dragging heavy freight had punched deep holes in the trail. For years, the horse teams had been the bane of the dog rigs. Back in 1900, one stampeder described how horses could wreak havoc on a trail:

[They] broke through every step, and it was the hardest riding I have ever seen . . . they would twist 8 foot sections right out of the trail. Most of the dogs had broken many of their toenails off having caught them on the edges of these horse tracks and holes. The trail was bloody for miles from the bleeding and limping dogs. . . . Many men had sprained their ankles and were limping. . . . What those dog men said and thought about the two men and horses would burn up a ton of asbestos fireproof paper.

Shannon's team fought to keep its footing, but finally Shannon accepted that the trail was too broken up to be of use. Shouting, "Haw!" he ordered Blackie to turn left and lead the team onto the Tanana River. The temperature would be several degrees colder on the frozen river than on the steep bank but at least the path had not been broken up by the horses.

Shannon was taking a big risk. In any type of weather, traveling over a frozen river can be extremely dangerous. River ice is in a constant state of transformation. It can be smooth along one stretch and a jumble of craggy ice sculptures on the next. The large frozen peaks are strong enough to support a truck, but the narrow valleys in between can easily crack underfoot.

It was nearly pitch dark, and though Shannon was fighting the numbing cold, he had managed to stay alert, and was watching for hazards along the river. He was particularly worried about overflow, a phenomenon that can occur in any type of winter weather, but which at 50 degrees below is life-threatening. Overflow occurs when water bursts through the surface and seeps over the top of the ice. The pent-up water can be under such pressure that it forms a geyser sometimes three or four feet high and the slick may spread for miles across the ice.

In warmer weather, many sled dogs love to splash through overflow, but in temperatures below zero a dog will do his best to avoid it. If a team drives through overflow in the bitter cold, a driver must stop immediately, cut down boughs of spruce, and build a fire to dry his moccasins and socks. A delay could cost him his toes, his foot, or his life.

It is also important to dry off each dog's paws, because the ice could build up and grind away at the pads, eventually crippling the animal. It was a cold and time-consuming operation that required working without gloves, but it was an absolute necessity. "A man is only as good as his dogs when he is on the trails of Alaska . . . and a dog is only as good as his feet," a well-traveled dog driver once said.

Overflow refreezes quite rapidly, forming a fragile shell that will crack loudly or flex like rubber underfoot, either of which are clear signals for the traveler to get off. But once the overflow has completely frozen to a hard sheen, it can be as slippery as glass and unyielding to any toehold.

The other risk of riding over frozen rivers was what has been described as drum ice, the opposite of overflow. This threat was the greater of the two: while a good lead dog could avoid overflow, he was often unable to detect drum ice in time to avoid catastrophe. Drum ice occurs when the water beneath a frozen river recedes, leaving behind a deep ice cavern. It appears quite ordinary on the surface, but when a team drives over it the sled begins to make a hollow sound, like a drum. If the team doesn't get off quickly the ice could cave in and the driver fall 10 to 20 feet down to the dry riverbed.

Either way, it would be important for Shannon to remain calm: if he panicked, the dogs were likely to sense it and become unnerved, and this would only worsen the situation. In most trail emergencies, a driver was usually better off letting an experienced lead dog handle the problem on his own, without interference. On the whole, lead dogs—males and females—tend to be calm and confident by nature. They earn their position not by being more aggressive than their peers but by sheer intelligence.

In the early 1900s, Bert Hansen, a deputy U.S. Marshal in Alaska, patrolled thousands of miles of wilderness, and it was his job to bring in the frozen and the dead, the criminal and the insane. One day, traveling over a frozen river in the Interior, he fell through drum ice and became stranded in a "crystalline tomb" 12 feet deep and 150 feet wide. His lead dog, Tuesday, heard the crash, felt the sled suddenly go light, and circled back with his teammates to investigate. (Many teams would just have kept going.) The dog looked down the hole at Hansen, whined, and dug his paws into the edge of hole, "as if he were going to leap in and join me," Hansen recalled. Hansen and Tuesday had traveled this same trail several times and the marshal knew that there was a trapper who lived in a cabin about ten miles away. "So I waved my hand in that direction and ordered Tuesday to mush. He barked, turned his head the way I had motioned and looked down as though trying to read my mind," and then took off with the dog team.

The minutes ticked by slowly and Hansen, now alone, began to panic. He grabbed at the boulders, hoping to pry them loose from the frozen gravel and stack them up against the wall to create a makeshift ladder. He paced the length of the cavern, found a place where the wall sloped, and realized he could cut toeholds in the ice and climb out. He patted his parka with his hands, looking for his knife. He had forgotten to pack it, a serious oversight. In despair, Hansen began to pound on the ice. "I was in one of those strange panics a man sometimes gets into when he finds himself absolutely up against it— Another musher had made his last mush, that was all!"

The trail-hardened driver fell to his hands and knees and started to scrape at the boulders until his fingers were bleeding. Managing to pry one stone loose, he repeatedly banged against the ice until he could finally claw his way out. Just as he was pulling out, Tuesday appeared around the bend with the team and the trapper on the runners of the sled.

"Do you wonder—I don't—that Alaskans called Tuesday my 'brains,' that they said it was only because of him that I was able to make some of the mushes I made?"

So far, Shannon had been lucky. His team had avoided any drum ice or overflow and the pups were working well together. But as the hours passed, a chill crept deeper into Shannon's bones. It was becoming harder and harder, he realized, to warm his extremities. He had to take immediate action and so began to swing his arms violently downwards at the same time that he began to pedal more frequently on the runners, hoping to drive the blood back into his fingers and toes. Then there was a gradual shift in perception. His focus began to move from the trail and the dogs to his own inability to stay warm.

Suddenly, Blackie made a sharp turn. The swing dogs followed in unison and the sled veered off. Shannon momentarily lost his balance but managed to hold onto the handlebars and regain his footing. Blackie's behavior had been odd, was Shannon's first thought, until he was able to piece together what had happened: Blackie had avoided a black hole, an opening in the ice that had been eaten away by the current underneath and was "large enough to drag down the entire team."

Blackie had either seen the steam rising off the river or heard the rush of current against the hard-packed ice. He may have even felt the first vibration of cracking ice beneath his feet, for black holes have a tendency to widen quickly. Either way, he had reacted quickly. But something was wrong with four of the pups. Bear, Cub, Jack, and Jet were no longer running steadily. Sled dogs, at their best, will place their back leg inside the print of their forepaw, and many of them will be in step with each other. But as dogs tire, they fall out of rhythm. A pair of hind legs will be slow on the uptake. Another dog will begin crabbing, leaving paw prints at the edge of the trail as he stumbles, lags, and has to be dragged forward by the other dogs. Cub, Jack, and Jet were clearly exhausted. They had nothing left to draw on but heart, the sheer will to keep moving forward with the other dogs. And Bear was not much better. Shannon had been on the trail for four or five hours now. The temperature was still dropping and the colder it became, the slower time seemed to pass.

Shannon's own physical problems had not resolved themselves, and worse, his attempts to get blood down to his extremities no longer seemed to be paying off. If he did not do something quickly to get more heat to his legs, he knew what would happen. He would die, along with his dogs, and perishing with them would be any hope of getting the serum to Nome. His body was simply losing heat faster than he could produce it. In an attempt to protect against the cold, his body was shunting blood from its extremities to its core vital organs.

Already his face was growing numb, and one of his big toes had become frozen. As sluggish as he felt, he knew what he had to do.

Shannon stopped the team and got off the sled. He raced to the front, just ahead of Blackie, and began to jog. The dogs matched their pace to Shannon's. When finally he felt the blood returning to his limbs, Shannon knew he had warmed up enough to go back to the sled and ride the runners.

This worked, but only for a while. Shannon was getting tired again, and, as he would recall, he was becoming "fairly stupefied by the cold."

He knew, as would any seasoned musher, what was happening to him: he was becoming hypothermic. A human being can shiver for just so long. The process is physically exhausting. It makes the muscles tense from the buildup of lactic acid and carbon dioxide. Soon it would be difficult for Shannon to hold onto the sled, let alone lean forward and pedal from the runners. With the loss of muscle control, his skin would grow pale, numb, and waxy. The uncontrollable fits of shivering would soon lead to stumbling, then to slurred speech, then mental lapses: moments of time unaccounted for, a wandering of the mind, odd behavior. A person suffering from hypothermia may even feel hot and begin taking off his clothes. Or lose the trail and begin walking in circles, unaware that he is stepping over his own footprints in the snow. Finally, apathy and exhaustion set in. A person will no longer care about reaching his destination. All he wants to do is to sleep. This feeling will nag him every step until at last he gives in to the desire, curls up in the fetal position, and closes his eyes.

At this stage, the body shuts down. All blood flow to the extremities stops, the breathing rate slows, and the pulse becomes shallow and weak. The victim is in a hibernation mode. The skin becomes bluish-gray and the limbs grow rigid. As the internal temperature continues to drop toward 86 degrees, the body becomes a metabolic icebox. To an observer, the victim will appear dead. It would be hard to find a pulse or see an indication of respiration. If the victim is in a fetal position, one specialist recommends forcing the arm to extend. It if curls back, the person is still alive. Only live muscles contract.

But in Alaska, where travelers are few and far between on the trail, hypothermia victims are rarely rescued from their deadly sleep. Men have been found encased in ice where overflow crept up around them as they slept. Others have been found sitting on a sled or on top of a boulder or frozen solid in the act of trying to strike a match.

Although death by hypothermia was relatively painless, the "long conscious fight" against a relentless chill could be agony for any experienced outdoorsman. As the traveling missionary Hudson Stuck once observed, "All of us who have traveled in cold weather know how uneasy and apprehensive a man becomes when the fingers grow obstinately cold and he realizes that he is not succeeding in getting them warm again. It is the beginning of death by freezing."

Shannon was losing track of time. He forced himself to focus on Campbell's roadhouse in Minto, where he could warm up. As Shannon raced toward Minto, he was no doubt aware of the danger he and his dogs were in. But there was nothing he could do except thrash his arms against his sides, stomp his feet when he could, and continue to jog ahead of the dogs for short periods. When his extremities failed to warm up even after these attempts, he knew there was not enough heat in his core to spare. With the fear building inside him, he pushed on, knowing he had to reach Minto before he lost control of himself and his team.

At around 3:00 A.M., the door to Johnny Campbell's roadhouse opened. Campbell took one look at Shannon and his dogs and it was clear to him that something terrible had happened. Parts of Shannon's face had turned black from severe frostbite. Blood had stained the mouths of Bear, Cub, Jack, and Jet. Helping Shannon inside, he placed him near the sheet-iron stove and poured him a cup of hot black coffee. Shannon was too tired and cold to eat. As he attempted the first sips from his coffee, he took a look at the thermometer outside: it was minus 62 degrees.

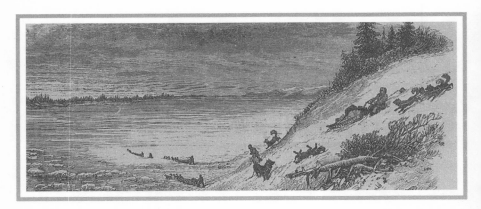

A nineteenth-century explorer's illustration of Athabaskan travel along the
Yukon River, the central highway of Alaska's Interior.

8

Along the Yukon River

"There are a few lonely places in this world, and the wastes of the great Alaskan Interior are the loneliest of them all."
— TRAVELER HENRY W. ELLIOTT, 1886

FOR FOUR hours, Bill Shannon sat huddled at the stove in Campbell's roadhouse, drinking coffee and allowing the heat to wash over him. Finally, he was ready to take some food to give him the strength to continue the journey. Despite all that had happened, Shannon had not lost his resolve. He would complete the remaining twenty-two miles to Tolovana. He had given his word that he would.

As Dr. Beeson in Anchorage had instructed, Shannon had taken the serum inside so it would not freeze, unwrapping the layer of fur and canvas and dangling the container from the rafters above to share the warmth of the stove. The cabin was probably no warmer than 50 degrees, but in comparison with the temperature outside it felt tropical. Just before seven o'clock on Wednesday morning, now working on his sixth cup of coffee, Wild Bill took a last pull from his cup and went outside to check on his dogs. Although by the clock it was early morning, it would be several more hours before dawn finally drove out the darkness of the Alaskan night.

Earlier that night, after helping Shannon into the roadhouse, Johnny Campbell led the dogs to a lean-to, where he fed them and let them rest. But one look suggested that they needed far more than an hour or two of downtime. Several were suffering from what mushers in those days described as "lung scorching," a condition in which they believed a dog's lungs were turned black as coal from frostbite. Lung scorching was more conjecture than proven fact. Mushers rarely, if ever, performed autopsies on their dogs and only imagined the havoc the cold air was causing them. Modern veterinarian medicine tells us that a dog suffering from working too hard in the severe cold more likely has a pulmonary hemorrhage. Sustained heavy exertion in dry, minus-50-degree weather can freeze and burst the minute vessels of a dog's bronchial tree and damage the delicate alveoli, the tiny sacs in the lungs where the transfer of oxygen to the blood takes place. The lungs do not turn black, but fill up with blood. Although the dog finds it harder and harder to breathe, he will keep running, spurred on by his teammates, until eventually he drowns in his own blood or passes out from oxygen deprivation. In either event, he will soon be dead. The initial warning signs are bleeding from the mouth and nose, where the lining of mucous membrane becomes brittle and cracks in the cold.

When Shannon checked on the dogs, Cub, Jack, and Jet could barely struggle to their feet. The trip to Tolovana was at least another three to four hours and Shannon knew that these dogs would not make the distance. He would leave the three behind. It was questionable whether they would ever run again, but at least for now he could take comfort in the fact that Campbell would take good care of them until he returned for them.

Down to six dogs, Shannon could only hope there would be no further mishaps on the trail. But Bear too was looking weak. He decided to let him try to make the rest of the run. If he had to, Shannon would take Bear off the team and put him in the sled basket. After readying the dogs, Shannon released the sled brake. The drive to Tolovana had now resumed.

THAT SAME morning, more than six hundred miles away at the other end of Alaska, the telephone rang at Leonhard Seppala's cabin at Little Creek, near Nome. It was the call Seppala had been waiting for. On the other end was Mark Summers, Seppala's boss at the Hammon

Consolidated Gold Fields and the man who had suggested Seppala for the western half of the relay. It was time, he was told, to head out.

Seppala was not a man to leave things to the last minute. That was how you got into trouble. Salmon for the dogs had already been stacked and tied down in the sled. Earlier in the week, Constance had frozen individual servings of precooked beans, ground beef, and hardtack that he could unwrap quickly and warm up on the trail for his own nourishment. All in all, he was traveling light; he had to if he wanted to make good time.

Seppala hung up the phone and put on his fur parka and mukluks. Out in the kennel, the dogs had heard the phone and were keyed up by the time Seppala stepped outside. When he headed toward them, they exploded in a frenzy of howls and yelps. They knew that it was time to run.

In the yard outside the kennel, Seppala laid out twenty harnesses. It was not easy to line up a team. Sled dogs usually become hysterical when they watch their teammates being taken out of the kennel for hooking up. This hysteria moves through the dog yard like electricity.

To get the job done, a driver must grab each dog by the collar and be dragged out of the kennel, all the while trying to steer the dog to his position on the team. He must then straddle the dog, which is leaping and yelping with excitement, and slip the web harness over his neck and pull his two front legs into the proper holes. Even in harness, the dog will jump back and forth over the gang line, getting necklines and tuglines tangled up with those of his teammates. Others will leap out at the driver for an extra pet or the chance to play for another minute, and they will surge forward to try to blow the brake and get the sled moving down the trail. Chaos and carnival.

Seppala understood that Nome was depending upon him and his lead dog, Togo. He not only had the longest leg to travel—315 miles to Nulato and 315 miles back, a journey of about six days—but one of the most difficult: the windswept ice of Norton Sound. There was also the probability of a blizzard delaying his journey, or worse, the ice breaking up and carrying him out to the sea.

The uproar in the kennel could be heard for miles around, and by the time Seppala had hooked up all the dogs, a small group from Little Creek had gathered to see the driver off. Seppala said a personal good-bye to his wife and to his curly-haired daughter Sigrid, mounted the runners, released the brake, and clucked. With the temperature at 20 below and the winds in a rare state of calm, the conditions were perfect for mushing. The dogs burst down the main trail in a sprint for Nome, three miles away.

Dog teams were hardly uncommon in a town where the mail was delivered by dogsled on a regular basis, but this twenty-dog team was a most extraordinary sight. As they raced toward Nome with their light load, the dogs barely skimmed the surface of the snow. They moved with a smooth, elegant gait, each tugline pulled taut, the gang line nearly strumming from the pressure.

Seppala shouted out commands from the back of the sled: with twenty dogs running at stop speed, he would be on the verge of losing control, but Togo responded to the commands as if he were attached to invisible reins. A crowd had gathered to watch Seppala run through town and it cheered mightily as he approached. Stray dogs darted up to the team and added to the general clamor, barking and nipping at each other's heels. The team careered around the sharp bend onto Front Street, with the sled bouncing and the bells on the handlebars jingling.

For this brief moment, Nome seemed to have returned to the glory days of the All Alaska Sweepstakes. When Togo reached the east end of Front Street, he darted through a passageway of shacks and out onto the beach trail. Soon, Seppala's diminutive outline faded into the distance and the crowd fell silent in the midmorning chill.

The weight of what lay ahead had begun to sink in.

EVER SINCE Billy Barnett's death eight days earlier, both Dr. Welch and his nurse Emily Morgan had had little time for sleep. Billy's five-year-old sister Katherine had also developed symptoms and even after receiving 15,000 units of the old antitoxin showed few signs of improvement: her throat was still lined with membrane. Over on the Sandspit, the Stanleys were struggling to keep the remainder of the family intact after the tragic loss of Bessie. The parents, Henry and Anna, and another daughter, Mary, had improved after receiving serum, but Dora had not. And now a neighbor, Minnie Englestad, was ill and required 2,000 units of serum. She got it, but at the expense of other patients. In town, both Mr. Cramer and Mr. Hillodoll had raw sore throats, but Welch thought it wise to see whether there was any improvement before using up more of his dwindling supply.

Welch and the other elders of the town knew there was good reason to be hopeful. The mushers had come through before under trying circumstances, and with Seppala's aid, surely they would come through again. But never before had so much been at stake, and it was difficult to keep up one's spirits knowing that the coldest weather in twenty years had already shut down regular mail service in Fairbanks and several parts of the Yukon Territory. It was only a matter of time before the bad weather reached Nome. There had been too many days of calm wind and clear skies and the town was overdue for a winter storm. Residents could only hope that the drivers made it to Nome before the worst of the winter weather closed off all access.

For Seppala and his team, there were no distractions yet. Now that they were out on the trail, the adrenaline was pumping and the rush that the dogs set out in would not wear off until they stopped for the night. On day four, Seppala and his dogs would be at Isaac's Point and there they would have to make what might well turn out to be the most important decision of the run: whether to cut across Norton Sound, running the team over the more dangerous form of sea ice, or take the safer coastline route around the inlet that was at least twice as long. The end point of both routes was the settlement of Shaktoolik, located on the southern coast of Norton Sound. From there, Seppala would pick up the mail trail to Unalakleet and then head over the Nulato Mountains to the Yukon River.

Time was important, but so was safety. The sound was known throughout Alaska for its treachery; many drivers avoided it. The ice was prone to sudden breakups and over the years it had taken more than its fair share of victims. Summers had warned Seppala not to risk crossing it.

Seppala had never given Summers his word. With Togo at the head of the team, Seppala had crossed Norton Sound several times in his career, though there were times when he thought he would never make it alive to the other side. But there were risks in delaying the arrival of the serum even by a day. When he reached Isaac's Point, he would have to read the ice carefully and make his decision. And he knew that much of that decision would depend on the actions of Togo, who, like many lead dogs, had a sixth sense when it came to danger.

A good lead dog is the brain behind every team. He (or she) is the smartest dog in a master's kennel as well as among the fastest and hardest working. The lead dog sets the tone. He has the power to demoralize a team by allowing his tugline to run slack or to inspire it by pulling hard and steadily through a dangerous spot on the trail. Lead dogs are generally calm and confident and have an innate understanding that they do not necessarily work for the master but with him, for the good of the team.

The position of lead dog is not for the fainthearted. A dog may have all the qualities generally associated with leadership—speed, intelligence, and dependability—but be unable to handle the pressure. A dog who doesn't want the position will let his feelings be known. He will turn his head from left to right repeatedly on constant alert for an exit away from the dogs chasing him from behind. Or just stop short, cower, and cause the team to collapse like a sock being turned inside out. It takes a large measure of courage, strong will, and an almost Zen-like quality of mind for a dog to make a good leader. They are the ones who must keep a straight course along featureless sea ice that seems to have no horizon, or face a blizzard head-on. They are also the ones who must make the decisions in an emergency and, maybe most important, know when to disobey a bad command, no matter how forceful a driver may be.

"It is absolutely almost impossible to place a price on a good dog, especially if he is a leader," said Olaf Swenson, a trader and hunter in

Siberia, who had helped Seppala import huskies to Alaska. "Buying one is almost like buying a human being who is to undertake a joint venture with you. You know that before your trip is over, the dog may have saved your life by his intelligence, instinct and courage.

"It is [the lead dog] and his team who will often lead you through a snowstorm when every guide . . . you have has failed. Many a time when I have been on the trail, fighting my way back to camp through blinding, driving snow I have turned the job completely over to the dogs; they could smell the way back to camp, pick up on an old trail which even a Native would be unable to find, and bring me safely in. Sometimes, when you are traveling on ice and the sled breaks through, a good leader who minds instantly and accurately will get you out without difficulty, whereas a poor one will simply increase your hazard and, likely as not, send you to your death. This is the kind of dependability on which it is impossible to place any market value. You try to find the animals you want, that you can believe in and depend upon, and once you have found them, you buy them (if you can) for whatever price you can arrange."

In Alaska, trail-hardened lead dogs had become the stuff of legends. And Togo was a living one.

By 1925, Togo was as well known in Alaska as Seppala. He had been the driver's leader for at least the past seven years and had traveled across every terrain imaginable.

On the face of it, Togo did not look like a great leader. He was small, about 48 pounds, with a black, brown, and grayish coat that made him look mottled, even dirty. He had won speed races and led the team on nearly every important expedition made by Seppala. At twelve years of age, Togo was still surprisingly fast, strong, and alert. He was the best dog Seppala had at navigating sea ice and would often run well ahead of the team on a long lead in order to pick out the safest and easiest route across Norton Sound or other parts of the Bering Sea.

As a puppy, however, Togo's calling was not immediately apparent and he would have been consigned to the status of ordinary house pet if it had not been for his boldness.

Born in October 1913, Togo was the only pup in the litter. His mother, Dolly, was one of the original female Siberians which Lindeberg had placed in the Pioneer's kennels. His father was Suggen, Seppala's leader during the 1914 All Alaska Sweepstakes. Seppala paid little attention to Togo when he was born. He was small and had developed an ailment that caused his throat to swell, so he spent much of his infancy in the arms of Seppala's wife, who applied hot rags to soothe the dog's pain. Despite the close attention from Constance, or perhaps because of it, Togo became difficult and mischievous. Whenever Seppala tried to harness the team, Togo would dash out and nip the ears of the working dogs, sending them into paroxysms of frustration. He was, as one reporter once wrote, "showing all the signs of becoming a full-fledged canine delinquent."

By the time Togo was about six months old, Seppala had given him away to a woman who wanted a house pet when she returned to the states. Togo, who had been named after the Japanese admiral who won the Russo-Japanese War, rebelled at his civilized surroundings. The more his new owner coddled him with steaks and attention, the more irascible he became. Within a few weeks, Togo had escaped, leaping through a windowpane and running several miles back to his mates at the kennel. Seppala took him back. "A dog so devoted to his first friends deserved to be accepted," he would later recall.

For the next several weeks Togo continued to get loose and harass Seppala's team when they hit the trail. His antics amused, infuriated, and intrigued Seppala. He noticed that whenever Togo met an approaching team on the trail, he would dart up to its leader and jump at him, as if he were trying to clear the way for his master. This behavior almost cost him his life. One day he ran up to a team of trail-hardened malamutes, got mauled, and had to be rushed by dogsled back to Little Creek. The experience would make Togo an even more valuable racing dog. One of the most difficult skills to teach a lead dog is how to pass another string without getting distracted and possibly lured into a fight. For the rest of his life Togo always kept a clear course, giving an oncoming team a wide berth. When he passed another team going in the same direction, Togo would lean into his harness, yelp, and speed ahead, leaving the opponent in his wake. "Like a lot of humans," Seppala said, "Togo had learned the hard way."

Togo was about eight months old when he finally found the opportunity to show his worth not only as a great sled dog but as a leader. One morning Seppala set out to a mining camp outside of Nome. He tied Togo up and instructed that he be kept secure for two days after his departure. He was in a rush. There had been a gold strike at Dime Creek 160 miles from Nome and a prospector had hired Seppala to get him there quickly. Seppala could not afford to have Togo hassling his team. The dog hated being locked up, and the same night Seppala left, Togo broke free from his tether and jumped the seven-foot-high fence surrounding the kennel, getting his hind leg caught in the top wire mesh. Hanging by his leg on the outside of the fence, Togo was "squealing like a little pig" until a kennel hand came out and cut the dog loose. Togo dropped to the ground, rolled over, and ran off after Seppala.

The dog ran through the night, followed Seppala's trail to the roadhouse at Solomon, and rested quietly outside.

When Seppala left the next morning, he noticed his team was off to an unusually quick start. He attributed it to the scent of reindeer somewhere ahead. But when he looked far off down along the trail, he saw a dog running loose. It was Togo. And Togo of course was up to his usual tricks. Throughout the day, he led charges against reindeer and bit playfully at the leader's ears. When Seppala finally caught Togo, he had no choice but to put him at the back of the team in the wheel position where he could keep a close eye on him. As he slipped the harness over Togo's neck, the dog settled down and became serious. He kept his tugline taut and his attention focused on the trail. Seppala was astounded. He finally understood what Togo had been wanting all those months: to be a member of the team.

As the day wore on, Seppala kept moving Togo up the line. By the end of the day, the eight-month-old shared the lead with a veteran named Russky and had traveled seventy-five miles on his first day in harness. It was a feat unheard of for an inexperienced puppy. This was no canine delinquent but an "infant prodigy," Seppala said. "I had found a natural-born leader, something I had tried for years to breed."

ALASKAN LITERATURE is filled with stories about natural-born lead dogs like Togo who saved their teams through an almost uncanny ability to size up obstacles. Without such dogs, many Alaskans believe, Alaska could not have developed.

One story about the steely nerve of a lead dog tells of Hurricane, a tough malamute owned by an Athabaskan Native named Black Luk. Black Luk was driving a team of fifteen huskies across Eyak Lake in the Interior one day in late April with a load of more than $100,000 in gold bricks and a ton of furs and other freight. It was a warm spring day and the team had been traveling for several hours. Luk had to cross the seven-mile-long lake in order to make his destination on time. The lake was firm as Hurricane trotted out onto the surface, yet the dog was cautious in his gait, keeping his nose low on the surface. About a mile out, Black Luk became worried and looked back. Water was seeping into the tracks left by his runners. The farther out the team traveled, the deeper the tracks became.

It was too late to stop the dogs and turn around. The sled weighed too much and would break through the ice if he did. Hurricane knew the danger they were in. Black Luk spoke to him calmly, not wanting to interfere with the dog's concentration. "Steady, Hurricane; but speed up a little if you think best. Looks to me like the only way we can keep this sled on top of Eyak is to keep it moving pretty lively." Hurricane wagged his lowered tail but kept his eyes glued to the snow beneath his feet. He kept his pace steady and the trail behind him straight. Not a dog shirked the tugline when their paws became wet with water seeping up from below. Then, almost imperceptibly, Hurricane picked up speed, causing the runners to glide higher on the snow. The other dogs followed.

Up ahead, Black Luk saw a mile-long depression in the snow's surface. They were in the middle of the lake. Black Luk held back the impulse to tell Hurricane to stop. As the team hit the rim of the depression, Hurricane "gave two sharp yelps and pulled the team into a dead run." Each dog jumped into his collar. The sled hit the lowest spot, slowed as the runners sank well beneath the wet snow and the sled became twice as heavy. Hurricane did not look back but pulled harder. As they pulled out of the depression, Hurricane gradually slowed down to a trot, his nose still down between his fore paws. "More gradually than any human orders could have accomplished it he had them back again in that steady even rhythm of a pattering trot."

When the team finally reached the other side of the lake and was on the safety of the shore, Black Luk looked back and "as far as the eye could see those sled runners were as straight as if they had been laid out by a surveyor's transit." If Hurricane had panicked, Black Luk, his team, and his gold would be at the bottom of Eyak Lake.

In the early 1900s, leaders and their teammates were highly trained from an early age and exposed to a variety of tasks, which improved their capacity to learn and adapt. A driver may use the same team to haul passengers, guard supplies, race, run a trapline—which requires stopping and starting and long rests—and simply to haul packs on their backs. The same teams were used to cross sea ice and run through the dense boreal forests of the Interior. One musher even spoke of how he taught his lead dog to bring wood in from the pile when the stack by the stove went low. Today, many teams are specialized. They either run sprints or the long-distance races such as the Iditarod or Yukon Quest. A driver could have about one hundred dogs in his kennel, whereas in the past drivers had at the most about thirty-five, allowing for more individual attention and exposure to a wider variety of situations.

In some situations, it is instinct rather than experience that counts. One such incident involved Dubby, the lead dog of sweepstakes racer Scotty Allan. While walking ahead of the dogs across a lake, Allan broke through the ice and went down into the water over his head. The walls of ice around his hole were thick enough to keep the current from dragging him under, but Allan could not crawl out. He began to shiver and called out to Dubby. If the dog could get close enough, he could grab his harness and be pulled out. Dubby edged toward Allan, but each time he got too close, the dogs behind backed up in fear. Dubby changed tactics. He restarted the team and headed away from the hole, and for a second Allan thought the dog was leaving him. But then Dubby "crossed the ice on the big crack at a safe place below me, circled around back of me, keeping as close to the hole as the other dogs would let him. Then it dawned on me what he was trying to do!" Dubby was running as fast as he could at an angle so that when he veered away from the hole, the sled would swing toward Allan. On the second try, Allan gave the command so that the sled swung close. Allan grabbed a runner and was pulled out.

"You can't tell me that dog doesn't reason," said Allan. "I'd have been in that lake yet if Dubby hadn't figured out just how close he could bring his team without their balking on him. . . . He was the greatest little general I ever had."

Many scientists are reluctant to attribute human emotions to dogs, calling it anthropomorphism. A musher will be the first to disagree. Sled dogs experience a gamut of emotions, particularly on long expeditions, and lead dogs are not immune. The job is both physically and mentally demanding and they often need a break from their responsibility. Heading back from an expedition, Norman Vaughan, a polar dog driver in the late 1920s and 1930s, noticed that the harness of his lead dog, Dinty, was slacking. A slack harness is unacceptable for a lead dog, particularly on an expedition. Vaughan decided to retire the dog to the back of the team and in his place harnessed a ten-month-old puppy who was quick to express his excitement over the promotion. As if he were ashamed, Dinty put his tail between his legs and hit the trail without one leap or excited yelp. At night, he hid his nose in his paws, looking at Vaughan and the other dogs with a forlorn expression.

After several days, Vaughan decided that Dinty had had a long enough break. The following day, Vaughan began to harness the dogs. He started with the wheel dogs, and as he moved up the line he stole a glance at Dinty. The dog was lying with his head on his paws, "pretending indifference." When Vaughan finally stood before the dog to put him back in lead, Dinty jumped up, "fairly trembling with excitement" to be back at front for the final pull home. "Who says a dog doesn't think, doesn't understand, has no pride of position?" wrote a dog musher on the expedition who had watched the whole affair. "They would have had their opinions reversed in short order if they could have seen Mr. Dinty step off on that journey. Head erect and sensitive ears pointing, his eyes fairly sparkling and that great black plume of a tail waving wildly erect, Dinty was again a lead dog to stir a driver's pride."

This pride that many sled dogs "feel" toward their work, however, could have unfortunate consequences. One musher, a missionary of the Hudson Bay region, regretted that he did not show his dog a little more respect when it came time to retire his old leader. The missionary Egerton Young described how his lead dog, Voyageur, could not accept being usurped by a younger dog. Voyageur was getting old and it was time to groom a new leader. Without much explanation or preparation, Young put a new dog in Voyageur's position and put the old leader toward the back of the team. The dog became furious, chewing through his own harness and then through that of the new lead dog. Young mended the harnesses, reprimanded the dog, and restarted the team. Voyageur rebelled and rebelled. He turned wild and snapped at the heels of the dog ahead of him, as if trying to catch up to the new leader. Young checked him with a whip. "Thus completely foiled in this as in every other scheme his dog intellect could devise, Voyageur suddenly collapsed," Young wrote. Like a good sled dog, Voyageur continued the journey, but his usual "proud, eager, ambitious spirit was completely broken. His high head with that ever alert eye went down and the long tail tried to disappear between his legs." Seeing the dog's utter dejection, Young unhooked the new leader and replaced Voyageur, but it was too late. Voyageur's heart was broken. For the remainder of the trip Voyageur did not once wag his tail or turn his eyes up toward Young as he so often had.

Even an attempt to put him in the best harness decorated with ribbons and silver bells, which all the dogs were so fond of, would not lift

Voyageur's spirits. The night the team arrived at Young's cabin, Voyageur trudged out to the middle of the nearby lake. Beneath a full moon, he sat on the ice, moaning and howling. When the moon sank down to the horizon, Voyageur lay down and died.

ON WEDNESDAY, January 28, the first full day of the relay, the sun finally came up some 650 miles east of Nome at the roadhouse at Tolovana, Shannon's final destination. There was still no sign of Shannon. Among the regulars waiting at the roadhouse and warming themselves by the three big stoves was twenty-one-year-old Edgar Kallands. Half Athabaskan (on his mother's side), half Newfoundlander, Kallands was typical of many of the drivers in the Interior who had been forced, from the time he was a young boy, to rely on his own wits for survival. Kallands would take the serum from Shannon as soon as he arrived.

By his own definition, Kallands was a loner. Dogs had played a large role in his life and at times they were his closest friends. Growing up in a small village in the Interior, his best friend had been a puppy. There was simply no one else around. "He was my dog, or I was his dog. One or the other," he once said. "He was raised up with me." As he grew up, his affection for dogs became even greater. While most teams would run into the woods when let loose, Kallands's dogs always stayed close, certain as they were that they would receive his affection: ". . . when I go away and come back and they're waiting for me, I pet them all right away. I wouldn't just pet one and go on. I pet the whole bunch. Anytime I got up amongst them, they were all right around me."

As his regular job, Kallands worked as a musher for the Northern Commercial Company. The night before, at around 5:00 P.M., he had pulled into Johnny Campbell's roadhouse in Minto with the mail after chauffeuring an auditor for the NC Company from trading post to trading post along the Tanana and Yukon rivers. Their progress had been painfully slow because of the cold, and several times they had been forced to stop on the trail and light a fire. He had come to rest for the night at Campbell's place and had barely finished hanging up his wet gloves above the stove when the phone rang. It was Earl Parson, the NC Company's agent in Nenana.

"I want you to go back to Tolovana and wait there," he told the exhausted Kallands. "There's a diphtheria epidemic in Nome."

In a few moments Kallands had his gloves back on and hitched the dogs back up. Despite the temperature, which was nearly minus 60 degrees, he doubled back to Tolovana, a twenty-mile drive.

It had been an exhausting day: he arrived at around ten-thirty that night, having traveled more than 70 miles that day and more than 150 over the past two days. The dogs needed a few days off as much as he did. That would have to wait.

Now, twelve hours later, just around eleven o'clock in the morning, when the stillness outside the Tolovana roadhouse would usually be broken only by the occasional crack of a tree splitting in the cold or the extended clang of ice cracking under pressure, Kallands heard the pattering of dogs' feet and the rustle of runners gliding through the snow.

It was Wild Bill Shannon. As the team approached, Kallands and the roadhouse owner and his family all went out to help.

Shannon's face was still creased and black with frostbite, and his dogs looked for all the world as if they had been done in. Even the coming of daylight had done little to raise the temperature, which was now running at around 56 degrees below zero. For Wild Bill, the relay was finally over. He had done his part against tough odds, and done it well.

After allowing the serum to warm up at the roadhouse, Edgar Kallands was ready to start the next leg of the relay. He hopped on his 16-foot mail sled and as if on autopilot, released the brake and took off. His share of the relay, thirty-one miles to Manley Hot Springs, would be overland through thick woods on a trail that cut across a wide bend of the Tanana River. It was as difficult a part of the trail as any. Years later, in an interview with a reporter, he recalled his memory of the day and what had driven him: "It was 56 below, but I didn't notice it. We were dressed warm. We didn't have down, but I had a parky. It went below my knees, so the heat couldn't get out. You was always running or moving; your feet never got cold. . . . But what the heck? What do you notice when you're 20 years old? You don't notice a thing. I think about it now. How did I survive?"

Behind the roadhouse at Tolovana, as if it were a normal day on the job, the Signal Corps operator dashed off a message to Ed Wetzler in Nenana, the governor's man in charge of overseeing the relay. "Anti-toxin departed Tolovana 11 A.M." The relay was on its way again.

SHANNON TRIED to rest in Tolovana, but he had the fate of Cub, Jack, Jet, and now Bear on his mind. In a few days, he would return to Nenana with all four dogs in his sled. Cub, Jack, and Jet would die not long after his return. Shannon's own frostbite had been so severe that it would be weeks before he would once again be able to touch his own face with a razor and shave. Even then, it was a painful experience.

He told a reporter that he had done nothing out of the ordinary, that his animals deserved all the praise.

"What those dogs did on the run to Nome is above valuation. I claim no credit for myself. The real heroes of that run . . . were the dogs of the teams that did the pulling, dogs like Cub, and Jack and Jet that gave their lives on an errand of mercy. I can't tell you yet whether I'll be able to save Bear or not. He's in pretty bad shape, and it looks like I may lose him."

No record exists of Bear's fate. He may have survived, but in all likelihood he never ran again—a horrible fate for an animal that lived and breathed solely to run with its pack down a moonlit trail. Some dogs just won't accept being left out of the team and will howl and moan as the team leaves the yard. Sometimes they will sink into depression and die. Even those who accept their fate to sit by and watch the team leave always keep alive the instinct to one day run again.

"If ever their master comes to them with harness in hand," a modern-day musher wrote, "they will struggle on arthritic legs to ready themselves for the trail. There may be pain in their backs, but there is always hope in their eyes."

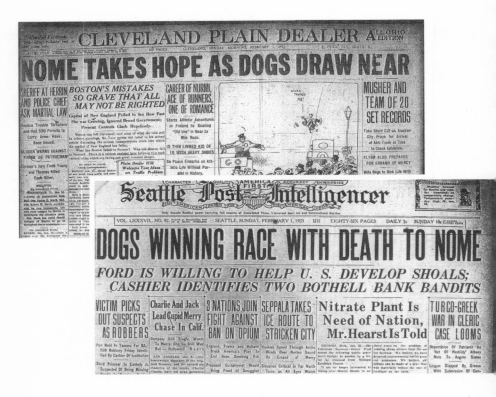

Headlines across the country told the unfolding drama in the far north
as the mushers drove their dogs across the Alaskan wilderness.

(Courtesy of the Cleveland Plain Dealer and Seattle Post-Intelligencer)

9

Red Tape

"Nome's Plight Worse: Nome Pleads for Airplane Relief Flight."
— *Seattle Union Record*

THE TEMPERATURE at Nome was 20 below, with a 10-knot wind blowing in from the north. In the dim purple light of the arctic morning, Emily Morgan and the other nurses who were gathered in the breakfast nook at Maynard Columbus Hospital could see the cross above St. Joseph's Church light up the sky like a constellation. Usually at this time of day, the staff would be finishing their breakfast, washing dishes, and taking the report of the night nurse coming off duty. But on this Thursday morning, January 29, the second day of the relay, there seemed little time for routine. The epidemic had taken a dramatic turn for the worse, and Welch needed all the help he could get over at the Sandspit and in town.

Yesterday had been another exhausting day; yet by that evening, after Welch and Morgan had examined their findings in preparation for their daily report to Mayor Maynard, there seemed some hope. Welch had been able to report to the mayor that no new cases had developed. It was a surprising discovery. Had the town turned the corner on the crisis even without new serum?

Unfortunately, it had not. Between late Wednesday evening and Thursday morning, at least two more children came down with diphtheria. One of them, Daniel Kialook, a Native on the Sandspit, had membrane covering both sides of his throat and a temperature of 99.6 degrees; another child in town was positively ill with diphtheria;

while several others were complaining of sore throats. Welch and Morgan now had some twenty confirmed cases on their medical list and almost double that number of suspected cases. Reports were coming in of at least one mother on the verge of a nervous breakdown, other parents in despair over the death of a child, and many more paralyzed with fear.

Now, Welch had to face the fact that he had no way of telling how many more cases would develop by the end of the day or in which quarter of town. Would he wake up tomorrow and find ten new cases or maybe even twenty? How many more parents at the Sandspit would Emily Morgan have to comfort as they buried their child? It was not the town population's fault. Both Native and white residents had obeyed the quarantine. Each full-blown case, as well as those suspected of having been infected, had been kept away from the general population. But the particular strain of diphtheria affecting Nome was simply too virulent for these basic precautions to make enough of a difference, and the lack of modern medical equipment to fight the disease was finally getting to Dr. Welch.

If only he had the means to perform the Schick Test. A little more than a decade earlier, in 1913, the Schick Test, named after the Hungarian-American pediatrician Béla Schick who created it, had been developed to identify those who had a natural immunity to the diphtheria toxin, most likely as a consequence of an earlier exposure that they survived. It was a simple test, an injection of diluted diphtheria toxin between the layers of the skin. If the skin turned red, the person was susceptible. With this information, Welch and Morgan would have been able to identify and then take special steps to shield those residents who were vulnerable and reassure those who were not.

Even without Schick Tests, Welch and Morgan could have reduced the severity of the epidemic and possibly brought it under control if they had throat swabs, a microscope, and an incubator for making cultures and identifying the presence of the bacteria. Although a person can be immune to the toxin the bacteria produces, he or she can still carry the bacteria and communicate it to others. In

addition, some people may take longer than others to develop symptoms or have such mild symptoms that their infection goes unde-
tected for days. Welch had no way of reliably distinguishing a child
with a nascent case of diphtheria from one who had a plain old sore
throat. Nor did he have a way of identifying healthy carriers and
preventing them from traveling freely, thereby spreading the conta-
gion, even beyond town.

Without these basic tools, the job of stemming the epidemic was
all the more overwhelming and time-consuming. Each sniffle and
cough had to be treated as if it were the start of the disease and each
healthy resident had to be looked at as suspect. And now the one tool
Welch did have, antitoxin—weak at six years old—was down to
21,000 units. From this point forward, Welch and Morgan would in
effect have to play God and determine who would receive the life-
saving medicine and who would not.

By early that Thursday afternoon, Welch passed on the news to
Mayor Maynard that his earlier, more positive assessment had been
premature. If the epidemic continued to spread at this new rate, there
could be several more deaths before the drivers carrying the 300,000
units reached Nome. "The situation is bad," a panicky Maynard
wrote in a telegram to Thompson in Fairbanks and Sutherland in
Washington; ". . . the number of diphtheria cases increasing hourly."
According to reports from the Signal Corps operator, the serum was
about 180 miles west of Nenana and was expected to reach Ruby at
around eight o'clock that evening. It was another four hundred miles
from Ruby to Nome; if all went well, it would be at least another
eight days before new antitoxin reached Nome.

Or would it? Maynard had never really given up on the idea of an
air rescue. Governor Bone had overruled him, not changed his mind.
With Welch's latest report and certain information he had recently
received from the governor, Maynard wondered if the time was ripe
to put in a second bid for a dramatic air rescue.

The previous day, Maynard had received a message from Bone
that more serum had been located in several towns near Juneau and
was being consolidated in the capital for shipment. This third batch

weighed about 12 pounds.[1] Bone was planning to send it by scheduled steamer from Juneau to the port town of Seward, where it would travel up the rail line to Nenana and wait for the next scheduled mail run.

Yesterday, the Juneau units had seemed minuscule compared to the 300,000 units en route and the 1.1 million units scheduled to depart by boat from Seattle on Saturday. But now, with the epidemic escalating, prompt delivery of even a 12-pound package might mean the difference between life and death for four to six terrified children who were at risk of slow strangulation. Now was the moment to turn up the heat a degree or two on Bone and on the federal authorities in Washington for an air rescue, and Maynard knew just the men to start the ball rolling—Thompson and Sutherland. Thompson, in particular, understood that if you wanted to get the full attention of Washington's politicians and officials, there was no better way than through the American press.

It had been easy to get their attention when the story first broke. From the day the Associated Press first reported the diphtheria epidemic in Nome and the dearth of antitoxin, the morning and afternoon papers, from San Francisco to Chicago to New York, had covered it without hesitation and in increasingly bold type. In a matter of days, Nome, Alaska, had once again captured the world's imagination, this time through a race of Alaska's dogs against the grim reaper. "Dogs Pitted Against Death in Nome Race," read the headline in the *San Francisco Bulletin*. "Dogs Carry Antitoxin to Snow Bound Alaskan City," wrote the *Washington Herald*. Editors fired off telegrams to Welch and Governor Bone, requesting exclusive interviews and personal accounts. Welch, with no time to spare, angrily declined. "I am a physician, not a press agent," he snapped. Bone on the other hand was, or at least had once been, a press agent. He typed out energetic reports

---

1. The serum was referred to only by its weight. Based on the weight of the 300,000 units—20 pounds—the serum being consolidated in Juneau was probably the equivalent of about 125,000 units, enough to treat about four to six patients.

for the International News Service praising the dog drivers, "who suffered for the sufferers" as they headed toward Nome.

From newspapers, the story soon jumped to radio. Audiences
across the country began to reach for the dial to tune in to the "Race
Against Death" taking place out there in the vast northern reaches of
the continent.

Soon it was not just Nome in the limelight. Towns forgotten
since the end of the Alaskan gold rushes once again became household names: Fairbanks, Tanana, Manley Hot Springs, and Ruby.
Men like Wild Bill Shannon, Edgar Kallands, and Curtis Welch
became symbols of America's thirst for adventure and for heroes.
Other news stories—a total eclipse over New York and a federal
war fraud case against former Assistant Secretary of War Benedict
Crowell—were relegated to sections below the fold, and everyone
from the lowliest official to the president himself had locked onto
the tale of the territory.

And then, as if nature herself were getting into the act, just as the
relay was starting, snowstorms and gales that had been battering
Juneau for days headed for the states, hitting the Midwest and the
Northeast from Maine to Georgia, pushing temperatures in New
York to record lows. The bad weather was killing people: in Elizabeth, New Jersey, a fifty-five-year-old man named Edward Sheridan
was found dead in a snowdrift just yards from his home. In Baltimore,
a nightwatchman in a stone yard froze to death near his shack. Harry
Kayhan of the Bronx collapsed from the cold at 41st Street and Park
Avenue. There were reports that children on their way to school had
been lost in the storm.

It was 1 below zero outside the warm apartments of New York,
and those looking out their windows were being given a small taste of
what living in the Arctic was all about. Manhattan had, ironically,
found itself icebound. The Hudson River had frozen solid, trapping
barges and ferries in ice floes. At the West 60th Street piers, two separate cargos of live cattle were unloaded and herded down Twelfth
Avenue to an early slaughter. The cows aboard were freezing to death
where they stood. There was havoc in the shipping lanes north and

train delays on the commuter lines. City and county workers in the thousands were trying to break up the ice and clear city streets.

A northeasterner unable to keep warm in zero-degree weather in New York could now begin to fathom what dogsledding in temperatures of minus 50 and 60 degrees might be like, alone and mostly in the dark of night. In living rooms across America, readers began drafting letters and poems in honor of the men and dogs taking part in the relay.

Maynard understood the intrinsic appeal of this man-against-nature story. He understood that the mushers were worthy of every bit of the praise and attention they were getting across the nation. But he also understood that Alaska desperately needed to move into the modern age.

The America of the 1920s was forward-looking, it was ebullient, but most of all it was an America captured by the belief that with a modicum of Yankee ingenuity, any problem could be solved. In the world of business, assembly lines and mass production were rapidly replacing the work of skilled artisans who might produce work of higher quality but at a cost only the very wealthy could afford. More and more Americans were trading in their horses and buggies for automobiles. Paved roads, built to accommodate fast-moving cars, were being laid down in every city and town across the country, and service stations providing food, gas, and "auto courts," the precursor to motels, were rising up across once lonely prairie land, their owners hoping to make a few dollars out of the new American wanderlust. Electricity too was reaching more and more households, and with the upsurge in available power came a concomitant interest in new appliances and technologies, such as the radio. As radio sets improved with the advent of new technologies that allowed for built-in speakers and AC power, Americans began to buy sets in great numbers. In 1922, some 60,000 households had a radio set; by 1924, there were more than 3.5 million.

Alaska needed to be part of this transformation. It needed modern communication and modern transportation, so that the next time an Alaskan town found itself without serum, or under threat from some different peril, it would not have to rely upon a Native technology that was older than anyone could calculate.

And there was something else driving Maynard, Thompson, and Sutherland. They were simply tired of being ignored by the federal government. After all, a good argument could be made that the federal authorities, having acquired Alaska, had in the end paid it little attention. Welch had asked for serum. His request had been ignored. In his annual report on the Yukon River region west of the town of Tanana, Governor Bone himself had observed that ". . . It is an unpeopled country, with abandoned mining camps bearing pathetic evidence of affluent days now gone, and steamers that once plied up and down the river beached at St. Michael and long out of commission. But for the boat service from Nenana to Holy Cross . . . this Yukon country would be wholly cut off from settled Alaska [the southeastern part of the state, especially around Juneau] and the outside world."

One could argue that there had never been enough people in the territory to justify the large expense of infrastructure needed to support a modern population; but one could also argue that new settlers were not going to come and make Alaska their home unless someone agreed to take up its cause and secured funds for roads and an air service. As it now stood, the 55,000 residents of Alaska had to take three separate means of transportation and travel over every terrain imaginable, up mountains, through forests, and over rivers, to reach the Interior from one of the towns of the southeast.

If it had to be a crisis in Nome that focused the nation on Alaska's plight, so be it. In an aggressive campaign of telegrams and exclusive dispatches, Maynard employed a no-holds-barred approach in the pleas he sent to wire services, newspapers, and institutions across the states, from the venerable AP and *The New York World* to the Seattle Chamber of Commerce.

"Help immediately!" Maynard begged in a cable to the AP.

Help by airplane with antitoxin serum is the appeal of Nome, not for sourdoughs, but especially for children of Young America of tomorrow.

We don't want to ask Russia to send an icebreaker with antitoxin, nor do we ask that the *Shenandoah* . . . be dispatched, but please get Uncle Sam to send a plane from Fairbanks where . . . men have volunteered to fly to Nome in four hours to bring relief to the dangerous situation prevailing here. Antitoxin shipped from Juneau would arrive in Nenana on Feb. 3, which if sent by airplane from there to Nome will beat the dog teams by several days, which may mean the saving of many lives.

Everything looked favorable yesterday but today conditions have been reversed. . . . Dr. Welch states . . . has only one good dose left and this is six years old.

There was no such evidence that the cases were mounting hourly, and Welch had more than one dose left, though not much more. But there was also no doubt that Nome was in crisis and Maynard's appeal eventually made its way to nearly every newspaper. Soon, his germ of an idea took on a life of its own.

"There is no denying that a well equipped airplane station with pilots and machines ready at a moment's notice to undertake an emergency journey is a crying necessity for Interior Alaska," said an editorial in Juneau's *Alaska Daily Empire*.

It is no longer a novelty, but becomes a part and parcel of modern advancement. Unfortunately it requires some catastrophe to awaken the public consciousness to some crying need. It required the *Titanic* tragedy to bring greater safeguards for the sea. It has required the diphtheria epidemic at Nome to awaken Washington to what [pilots] Noel Wien and Ben Eielson have been urging for two years. It is hoped that the costly lesson—the safety of Alaskan babies—will have gone home to bear fruit.

Soon, nearly every American newspaper printed Maynard's broadcast for help, publishing it on their front pages and giving it a prominent headline. *The Washington Post* urged that the "Epidemic Grows Graver, City Begs Officials Here to Send Aid by Air." In New York,

The Sun suggested that an air rescue would be "the greatest humanitarian service ever rendered by a flier in peace time," and the pilot Roy Darling became in the eyes of American public the "crippled war flier"—even though his crash had occurred after the war—who was willing to risk his life to race "over the icy wilds" to Nome.

Washington immediately began to reconsider its stance on the proposed mercy flight.

DELEGATE SUTHERLAND was the first politician to move into action. With the snow still thick on the ground in Washington, D.C., Sutherland approached the Justice and Navy departments for official permission for Roy Darling to fly a plane out of Fairbanks. Permission was granted. He then moved over to the U.S. Surgeon General and the Public Health Service and urged officials there to review the possibility of an air rescue to Nome. They were, it seemed, open to the idea.

Sutherland then wired Thompson and Mayor Maynard the good news. "Aviator Darling of Fairbanks has permission from Dept of Justice and the Navy Dept to make flight to Nome if required STOP Have just wired this information to Fairbanks STOP Keep me informed, official collect," Sutherland said in the message to Maynard.

For Sutherland, this must have been a moment of pure joy. An air rescue would not just further his dreams of establishing air-mail routes throughout Alaska but bring back from the edge of extinction a town that had so influenced his own life.

The news from Sutherland, however, did little to calm Maynard. By the following day, Friday, January 30, the mayor's anxiety had escalated. Apparently there had been another death overnight, bringing the death toll to five since the outbreak began on January 20.

Dr. Welch and Nurse Morgan were now monitoring twenty-two patients and thirty suspects. At least fifty-five people, according to his medical records, had been in close contact with someone who had the disease. Among the seriously ill was the young daughter of a miner named John Winters. She had membrane on both sides of her throat and a 102-degree fever. Welch gave her 6,000 units of serum, bringing his supply down to 13,000.

After hearing the day's tolls from the doctor and his staff, Maynard again hurried to the Signal Corps office, this time with a much more audacious plan. The chances were high, he knew, that even with the epidemic worsening, Governor Bone could not be persuaded to allow a plane to fly in the 12 pounds of Juneau serum. So Maynard decided to turn up the pressure a notch. He addressed his next telegram to his colleagues at the Chamber of Commerce in Seattle. He wanted Seattle businessmen to use their influence in Washington to prepare a plane to leave from Seattle with the 1.1 million units of the serum that were scheduled to leave on board the steamship *Alameda* tomorrow and head for Alaska's ice-free port of Seward. A plane could get the 1.1 million units of serum to Nome within seventy-two hours and wipe out the epidemic in its entirety.

The Seattle businessmen moved on the suggestion and wired the Chamber of Commerce's representative in Washington, J. J. Underwood, asking him to use his influence to secure a meeting with Major General Mason Patrick, chief of the U.S. Air Service.

The year before, the air service, with the help of the navy, had launched the first successful round-the-world flight on planes specifically built for long-distance flying. The planes were Douglas World Cruisers with 50-foot wingspans and cruising speeds of 90 mph that had been built by a torpedo-plane manufacturer, Donald Douglas, who worked out of an abandoned movie studio in California. On that epic round-the-world flight, teams consisting of a pilot and a mechanic set off in four separate aircraft from Seattle and flew up the Pacific Coast to Alaska and down the Alaska Peninsula to the Kuriles and beyond, circling the globe and touching down in Seattle five months and twenty-two days later. A major aim of the multi-stop expedition had been to provide U.S. pilots and their support crews with experience in the preparation and logistics of long-distance flying.

The chamber wanted one of those fliers, Lieutenant Erik Nelson—who had also been a member of the Black Wolf Squadron that had flown from New York to Nome via Fairbanks in 1920—to fly the serum to Nome. Nelson's chances of succeeding in a Douglas World Cruiser were far greater than Darling's chances in a flimsy aircraft of the Fairbanks Airplane Corporation.

The proposed flight, in which Nelson would take off from the Sand Point federal aviation field north of Seattle with Nome as his destination, would be a groundbreaking event: a rescue attempt that was also the longest air-mail flight in U.S. history.

The press understood the significance of the proposed flight and quickly called in experts to debate the possibility. Sand Point Commander Lieutenant Theodore Koenig, reached by the *Seattle Union Record* and the *Post-Intelligencer,* confirmed for reporters that a properly equipped plane with a large flying radius leaving from Sand Point could reach Nome before one of the smaller planes in Fairbanks. But if Maynard had hoped for a ringing endorsement from experienced fliers, he soon learned that he would get nothing of the sort. "Even so, the flight from Seattle presents grave difficulties as the opportunity to make favorable landings and replenish the fuel supply en route to the northern city is practically nil."

The longest single hop of the 1924 flight had been about 875 miles. Nome was more than 2,000 miles from Seattle. Furthermore, the U.S. War Deptartment had taken nearly a year to prepare supply depots and landing places, and to coordinate patrol vessels before the 1924 fliers embarked on their round-the-world journey. In addition, an army plane leaving Seattle in winter would have to be equipped with pontoons to make the trip from Seattle to Seward port and then refitted with skis for the overland journey to Nome. This alone, added Koenig, "would take longer, after preparations along the route had been made, than to transport the serum by dog team."

Major H. C. K. Muhlenberg, commander of the air service unit of the ROTC at the University of Washington, agreed. He added that any pilot flying to Alaska would need an electrically heated suit, and it would take time to track one down because none were currently available north of San Diego.

While the experts continued to debate the merits of the flight, one reader in New York and the general manager of a major U.S. wire service were working on an entirely different plan. The reader was Carl Lomen, son of the former Nome mayor, who was in the city on business. The wire service general manager was Loring Pickering of the North American Newspaper Alliance, an organization that had the power of sixty-nine newspapers behind it. Lomen and Pickering wanted Washington to take a greater role in the rescue effort and had come up with an idea that would solve the problems of refueling and landing. They wanted the government to send a cruiser with a plane on board up the Pacific Coast as far north as the Bering Sea ice line so that when the plane took off, it would have the shortest possible trip to Nome.

In a telegram to the U.S. Surgeon General, the Alliance offered to find and pay for a bacteriologist, culture tubes, swabs, an incubator, and other emergency laboratory supplies at any point on the Pacific Coast if Washington would dispatch a "cruiser carrying airplane and crew" to the edge of the ice pack of the Bering Sea. According to the telegram, the ice pack reached as far as Nunviak Island that winter, only some three hundred miles south of Nome.

In addition to the offer, Pickering's telegram gave space for the personal element of the tragedy unfolding and allowed Lomen to type in his own message. Lomen implored the Surgeon General to act immediately upon the Alliance's suggestion and

> not permit this epidemic to ravage our community as the influenza epidemic of 1918 unfortunately did . . . even successful delivery of antitoxin now en route by dog sled will by no means save situation. . . . Everything humanely possible should be done. . . . Even if the dog sleds should arrive within ten days, which would be a remarkably quick trip considering the possibility of Alaska blizzards, there would still be a need in Nome for a large additional quantity of serum and laboratory equipment. May we have immediate reply so no valuable time, meaning lives, is lost.

The telegram arrived at the office of the U.S. Surgeon General and got pushed all the way up to the desk of President Coolidge, who instructed his health czar to provide Nome with whatever it needed.

Sutherland, meanwhile, was continuing to pressure the War Department and the Surgeon General's office. The likelihood of a Seattle-to-Nome flight had diminished as the very real problems such a flight posed became more and more apparent. But what about the Newspaper Alliance's proposal? An aircraft carrier was a fairly new innovation. In 1921, the navy had set up its Bureau of Aeronautics and a year later had commissioned an old collier, the *Langley*, into an aircraft carrier with arrester gear. A landing platform only 534 feet by 64 feet was built over the deck and it could transport about fifty planes. It was nicknamed "the Covered Wagon" because the landing deck shaded the entire length of what had been the main deck. The ship had been the scene of several flying exhibitions and by 1924 had become part of the Pacific Battle Fleet operating off the California coast.

The navy had less than twenty-four hours to make its decision. It could send the *Langley* or it could send one of the fleet's battleships that had had the turret converted to launch a plane. Sutherland urged the bureau to take a role in the rescue, but by the close of day, the navy had decided that the trip was too risky. A cruiser would not be able to get close enough for a plane carrying serum to make a nonstop flight to Nome without itself risking being crushed by the Bering Sea ice. The best the navy could offer, it said, was to place its minesweeper *Swallow*, which operated along the northwest Pacific Coast as well as in Alaskan waters, on high alert to rush any bacteriologist and lab supplies found by the Alliance to the ice-free port of Seward.

"We have been conferring with Delegate Sutherland and public health officials about situation," the navy rear admiral said in his reply to Pickering, "and will render whatever aid possible."

At least one expert disagreed with the navy's decision: the explorer Roald Amundsen also happened to be in New York, and there he was attempting to drum up support for his 1925 aerial assault on the North Pole.

A cruiser was entirely feasible, he told reporters; "from what I know of the Western Coast of Alaska at this time of year, I am convinced that a cruiser or destroyer could get within firing range of Nome." As it turned out, the aerial flight to the pole Amundsen was planning at the time would be a disaster. The engines conked out en route. But that flight and its failure were still in the future. Despite the strong endorsement of one of world's most renowned explorers, the U.S. Navy still would not commit.

Sutherland kept up his lobbying efforts to fly the Juneau serum. Over the past two days he had kept one card close to his chest— William Thompson in Fairbanks. In the event that the War Department declined Maynard's plea for a plane, Sutherland had cabled Thompson to begin preparations for a flight: ". . . suggest aviator Darling have sourdough passenger who knows the trail," he told Thompson. "My suggestion to send snowshoes in event forced landing at a distance from the trail. Calm weather conditions reported on Bering Sea coast, maximum 19 below, north wind."

Thompson gathered up the crew of volunteer mechanics and ordered them to begin assembling the plane. He then went on a hunt for a mechanic to assist Darling during the flight and found Ralph Mackie, a resident of Anchorage who had flown with the Royal Flying Corps in Canada. Meanwhile, a former war pilot, who had been traveling in the Interior en route to Siberia to take photographs, learned of the epidemic, and sent a telegram to Thompson that he was heading to Ruby, a town along the mail route, where he would wait to help Darling refuel when he landed. Ruby had a depot of aviation fuel that had been left behind by the army for the pilots of the 1920 New York–to–Nome aerial expedition. The former war pilot could decant the fuel into canisters and be ready for a quick turnaround.

For the first time, the plane seemed a real possibility: the craft was being assembled and Darling now had an experienced co-pilot who knew the country. Even the temperature had warmed by 10 degrees, to minus 39. But they still needed to get control of the serum, or all these preparations would be for naught.

Thompson and Sutherland kept up the pressure on Governor Bone, urging him to approve the flight. Bone refused. They then turned to Edward Wetzler, the point man for the relay in Nenana, and pestered him to hand over the Juneau serum as soon as it arrived by train. Wetzler adamantly declined. His loyalties remained with the governor. Even the Surgeon General's office, which appeared to question Bone's decision, balked at ordering him around, requesting solely that Bone "use his discretion."

Once again, the *News-Miner* editor was livid. "Nome looks to Fairbanks for LIFE, and if there is not too much Red Tape interfering, Fairbanks will be in Nome in less than almost no time," Thompson wrote in his paper. ". . . Fairbanks is standing by, lashed to the mast . . . beating its Sourdough wings off trying to rush to the help of its friends, and restrained from doing it."

BONE REFUSED to budge. Despite immense pressure and a rising tide of calls from the press for a dramatic air rescue, he stuck with his decision, calling the proposition to dispatch icebreakers and cruisers to clear the way through the Bering Sea absurd and a flight that would overtake the dog teams even more so. Bone wired Wetzler, ordering him not to release the 12-pound package of serum from Juneau to anyone under any circumstances. The serum would stay in Nenana until a mail team could pick it up.

But no man rises to the level of governor without some measure of political skills, and if Bone understood anything, as an ex-reporter and ex-PR man, he understood public opinion. To do nothing but stay the course would subject him to the criticism of stubbornness at best, and a callous disregard for human life at worst. There was also the possibility that to do nothing would hurt Nome. If the epidemic was gaining ground at the speed Maynard had warned, the relay, Bone realized, had to be sped up.

Bone summoned his aide. He told him he wanted to call in more drivers for the final part of the run between Nulato and Nome for the 300,000 units of serum. And for this he needed the help of Mark Summers, the superintendent of the gold company in Nome.

The decision was both risky and shocking. In effect, Bone was risking cutting out the most important man of the relay—Leonhard Seppala. And he was asking Mark Summers, Seppala's sponsor, to do the cutting.

The argument for the change made sense. Although Seppala was the fastest driver in Alaska, under the original plan he had 630 miles round trip to cover. Even traveling light, Seppala still had to pace himself in order to survive. As fast as he was, no one man could beat fresh recruits who had to travel only a short distance before they turned the serum over to someone else.

But the change in plan did not take into account two very important factors. The first was that Seppala was still the best man to take the serum across Norton Sound, a dangerous shortcut but one that could save at least a day of travel. To preserve that part of the original plan, Seppala had to be informed that instead of driving all the way to Nulato, he should wait for the serum somewhere near Shaktoolik, on the southwest coast of the sound, for the oncoming driver.

The second factor was that there was no longer any way to communicate with Seppala. The telephone lines in Nome went only as far as Solomon, about thirty-five miles east of town. In addition, the Signal Corps system bypassed the villages along the coast by shooting across Norton Sound to St. Michael, where a relay station conveyed messages to Unalakleet and then up the Nulato Mountains and over the Kaltag portage to the Interior and beyond. While the new plan still assumed that Seppala would make the dangerous run back across Norton Sound, it relied upon the driver heading north to find Seppala. Two oncoming drivers could easily miss each other in blizzard-force winds. At times, the air was so thick with snow that one could not even see the large tripod stakes marking the trail.

Still, Bone's order had to be followed. Summers immediately tracked down Ed Rohn, a dog driver whose claim to fame was that he had once beaten Seppala in a race, and ordered him to drive twenty-one miles to Port Safety and wait there at the roadhouse for further instructions. He then called out to the kennels at Little Creek, got Gunnar Kaasen, another Hammon dog driver, on the phone, and requested that he put together a dog team and drive to the mining village of Bluff, about thirty miles east of Safety. Kaasen went to the kennels, looked over the team, and began to harness up the dogs that had been left behind. Before he left, Seppala had made it clear that if Hammon needed a team for company business, Fox, a brown-and-black-furred husky, should be the leader. Kaasen, who worked closely with Seppala at the gold fields in the summer, had apparently always admired another dog from afar. The dog was stocky for a Siberian, black as night except for a white right foreleg. His name was Balto. One by one, Kaasen brought the dogs to the gang line. When it came time to clip in the leader, he ignored Seppala's direction, and brought Balto to the position.

It was a decision that would forever leave a strain in the relationship between the two colleagues.

When Kaasen reached Bluff, he was to enlist roadhouse keeper Charles Olson, a bachelor and old-time sourdough, and tell him to hitch up his rig, drive twenty-five miles further east to the trading post at Golovin, and wait for the serum.

While the drivers prepared to take up their positions, Summers reached the storekeeper in Unalakleet via the Signal Corps system and told him to "spare no expense" in posting more teams on the trail. At least two more teams were placed, one in Unalakleet and another thirty-eight miles up the coast at Shaktoolik.

All told, 20 men and about 150 dogs would now be taking part in the race to save Nome. As for Seppala, all that could be done was to warn the new men on the route that in addition to carrying the serum toward Nome, they should keep a lookout for the Norwegian and his team of Siberian dogs. Should they meet up with Seppala, they were to stop him and hand the serum over to him. Summers had already calculated that the most likely place for a handoff would be somewhere near Shaktoolik.

With the new plans in place, there was little more that Bone could do but wait. It was probably clear to him that if the dogs failed, there would surely be hell to pay, given his stubborn refusal to allow a daring air rescue.

All Nome could do was also wait and perhaps pray that the

weather would continue to hold. Welch maintained his vigilance of the sick. By tomorrow, his supply would be exhausted. But he wasn't ready to give up. Later that day, Welch walked over to the Signal Corps and sent a telegram to his concerned sister back home. "We are working night and day," he wrote, "and are going to keep at it until we get the best of it."

Two DAYS earlier, on Wednesday, January 28, the young Edgar Kallands, who had taken the 300,000 units of serum from an exhausted Wild Bill Shannon, completed his run to Manley Hot Springs with relatively few mishaps. The weather had been a brutal 56 degrees below and, according to one newspaper report, Kallands's gloved hands froze to the sled's handlebar: the trip from Tolovana had taken more than five hours and the roadhouse owner had to pour boiling water on the birchwood bar to pry him loose. Kallands stayed overnight in Manley, and he and the dogs finally got the rest they needed. Then they began the fifty-four-mile journey to their home in Tanana, the geographical center of Alaska. At Tanana, Kallands and his fellow townsfolk would listen to the progress of the serum run by telephone over the old telegraph line between Tanana and Ruby that the Corps had abandoned when it went to wireless communications.

Names of fellow Athabaskans like Sam Joseph, Titus Nickolai, Dave Corning, Harry Pitka, and George and Edgar Nollner would crackle across the wire over the next two days as each continued the westward relay across the Interior to meet Seppala.

At 3:00 A.M. on Friday morning, January 30, Charlie Evans, the twelfth driver in the relay, was waiting at Bishop Mountain when he heard a dog team approaching in the distance. The driver was George Nollner, Evans's close friend, and he was humming an Athabaskan love song, thinking of the woman he'd married a few days earlier. George had split his run, between Whiskey Creek and Bishop Mountain, with his older brother, Edgar, in order to speed the serum down the trail. When George arrived, he unwrapped the package and the two went inside the cabin to sit by the stove and warm the serum. They stayed inside for nearly an hour, worried that the deepening cold would freeze the medicine and render it useless.

The temperature had warmed slightly over the past day. But it had been only a brief reprieve. By early morning, a troubling cold had begun to set in. Outside the cabin, when Evans looked up at the sky, the green and white lights of the aurora borealis danced a slow, graceful waltz. Like so many of the mushers, Evans was half Athabaskan on his mother's side. Descended from a long line of powerful Koyukon chiefs, he came from a tradition of helping people through times of need. For many Athabaskans, the northern lights were the torches of spirits to guide travelers on their journey to heaven. All one had to do was whistle, and according to their legend, the spirits would come down out of the sky to one's aid. But Evans knew not to be lulled into a false sense of security. The temperature was minus 62 degrees.

Evans's run would begin at Bishop Mountain, a fish camp on the north bank of the Yukon River. Here, the Yukon makes a sharp S-curve around a 200-foot pile of stone. Most years, the ice is rough and uneven, the tortuous leavings of immense floes that have crashed and sheared against the sudden turn in the bank, wrenching free avalanches of dirt and rock. Evans knew this stretch of the Yukon the way a gardener knows every flower in a bed, every twist and turn, and every shift in its sandbars and shoals. In summer, the twenty-two-year-old dog driver piloted a riverboat, navigating the Yukon and the nearby Koyukuk tributary, which tumbles down from the Brooks Range. The two rivers meet ten miles west of Bishop Mountain at Evans's home village of Koyukuk. His father, John Evans, a gold miner from Idaho, ran a store there, and in winter Charlie helped out his dad transporting merchandise and furs by dogsled.

IT WAS about 4:30 A.M. when Evans finally started off on the thirty-mile trip from Bishop Mountain to Nulato. He had been up all night waiting for George and was already slightly tired. Just ten miles into his run, he ran into trouble. The suppressed waters of the Koyukuk had broken through the ice where the river converged with the Yukon and covered the trail for half a mile with overflow. The dogs managed to avoid the open water, but the relative warmth of the vapor rising up off the river created a thick, cottony wall of ice fog. The fog rose to Evans's waist and swallowed the dogs and the sled.

Ice fog can be 30 to 60 feet thick and cover miles of ground. It creates a ghost world haunted by ice crystals shimmering and floating in the air, suspended like motes of diamond dust that part and close in when disturbed by a breeze or a person moving through it. Once into the fog, a driver can only feel his way over the trail. He has no way of gauging how far he has come or in which direction he is going. In this thick icy mist, no longer able to use the sight of a familiar trail to anchor him to reality, he can be overcome by a sudden sense of helplessness. "It would come over me all of a sudden," a driver once wrote, "a sort of helpless feeling, as if no matter how hard we struggled, we weren't getting anywhere . . . there were times out there that I thought I was going nutty."

Evans didn't dare get off the sled. He drove blind through the fog, grateful when the thick mist ahead of him lowered enough to reveal the tips of the dogs' tails and the bobbing tops of their heads. All he could do was stand on the runners, hold on for bumps, and "let the dogs go. . . ." Many dogs would balk in the blinding whiteness, but Evans's dogs "knew what they were doing. I trusted the dogs. They trusted me. They had a sixth sense, seemed to know what I was thinking." A light breeze had begun to blow, creating a wind chill, and Evans, on the back of the sled, began to stiffen up with the cold. The wind was blowing sand off the exposed portions of the steep bank; under such conditions the sand could feel like shards of glass when it hit a driver's face.

Evans's two lead dogs faltered, misfiring their gaits. They were mixed breeds, a combination of bird dog and husky, and Evans had borrowed them to fill out his own team. But they had more bird dog in them than husky and were ill suited for such difficult pulling. Their hair was short and the harnesses were beginning to constrict their legs and chafe. Worse, Evans had forgotten rabbit skins to protect the dogs' groin area, which has little hair, and the two of them had already begun to freeze as they ran.

Evans neared the village of Koyukuk where his father, John Evans, was waiting, straining for any sounds of his son. John heard the squeak of the runners against the cold snow and ran out to the bank to urge his son to stop, to come inside and warm up.

"I can't stop," Charlie had shouted back from the river. "Them dogs would be hard to wake up."

John Evans watched his son pull away. John had organized the drivers on this stretch of the Yukon, and when he told his son about the epidemic in Nome, Charlie did not hesitate to volunteer. Charlie's mother had died in 1908 when he was only five; John Evans then put everything he had into Charlie and his brother, teaching them the ways of the Yukon and sending them to Oregon to school for five years to learn the ways of the modern world.

Five miles past Koyukuk, the river swung 90 degrees to the south southwest and ran along a ridge of densely wooded trees which rose 1,000 feet above the river. Nulato was about ten miles away.

Some time after Charlie left his father behind, the legs of his two lead dogs turned blue and became swollen, burned raw by the cold where the harnesses had cut away the skin and fur. They had severe frostbite. The dogs stumbled on, until suddenly one of the lead dogs dropped to the ground. Then the other went down. The team stopped and Evans, chilled by the cold, staggered up to the front. Both dogs were crippled. Evans had no choice but to put both in the basket of the sled. According to one report, he moved to the front of the team, where he strapped a harness over his shoulder and helped the remaining dogs pull the sled over the last stretch of the trail to Nulato.[2]

2. The report does not make clear whether Evans said he had to move to the front of the team, and other sources make no mention of the issue. However, it is plausible that Evans had to take up the lead position, as he probably did not have another dog in the team capable of leading—or he would not have borrowed the two dogs. A swing or wheel dog cannot be graduated to the front position without proper training.

A little before 10:00 A.M., Evans could see the outline of Nulato Island in the middle of the river, and a little ways beyond, off to the right, was Nulato. As Evans pulled in to the village, he carried the lead dogs into the cabin and slumped by the stove. Both dogs were dead. When asked about the run some fifty years later, Evans simply recalled: "It was real cold."

THE SERUM had been on the trail now for three days and had traveled 356 miles to the original meeting point. But now they had been told to go further. There were still 318 miles to go and the job of moving the serum 36 miles closer to Nome now rested in the hands of an Athabaskan Indian called Tommy Patsy, who had made a distinctive name for himself a few summers earlier when he and two other men had been chosen by their elders to take part in one of the last hunts of a grizzly by spear. The Koyukon elders had known that this might be the last time a young hunter would take a bear by spear, because the tradition and the knowledge of the difficult task were rapidly dying out. Still, killing a grizzly by spear was considered among the Koyukon as the ultimate test for a man as well as a hunter.

Patsy and the others trained in secret all summer for the hunt, strengthening their muscles, running, and practicing the pole vault. In the hunt, Patsy and another of the hunters, Sidney Huntington, would vault over the den with dried birch poles and use the poles to keep the "big animal" trapped inside, while a third hunter, opposite the den, steadied his spear in a small hole in the ground. When he was ready, the others would lift up their poles and free the raging bear. To test their pole-vaulting skills, Patsy and Huntington had to vault over a big fire of spruce boughs in fur parkas. If the parkas burned, they would be disqualified. They passed, and later that winter they successfully killed the bear by spear, perhaps the last of their people to do so.

True to the tradition, Patsy never bragged about the hunt. To have done so would have brought bad luck upon his village. Nulato had had its share of troubles. The village was the site of a Russian fort and trading post in the Interior. In 1851, the garrison and most of the

Natives living around it had been massacred by a band of warring Indians. Patsy learned of the massacre from his elders, who passed the story down through the generations. Not infrequently, residents walking around the site of the fort found buttons from the uniforms of the Russian soldiers.

About half an hour after Charlie Evans arrived, Patsy secured the serum in his own sled and with the fastest dogs in the village set out on the trail, which followed the direction of the river southwest to Kaltag, a village that sat on a bluff overlooking the Yukon. At Kaltag, the trail left the Yukon River and headed over the mountains, where the weather grew worse. Kaltag was the start of the ninety-mile-long portage that linked the Interior with the Bering Sea coast. It began with a steep, fifteen-mile incline into the 4,000-foot Nulato Mountains before flattening out and descending to the coast. It was like a tunnel to a new, even more dangerous world. At the other end of the portage, at the Native settlement of Unalakleet, the relay would leave the relatively calm but cold Interior and enter the unpredictable conditions of the coast.

The serum had yet to face its greatest challenge—the crossing of Norton Sound.

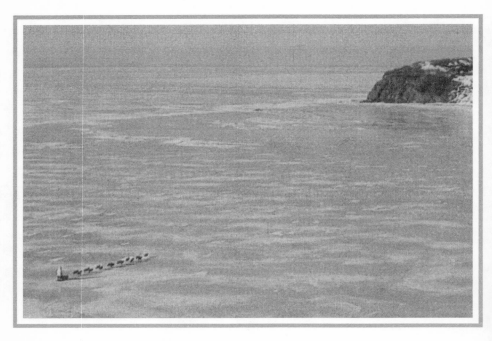

A dog team crossing the dreaded Norton Sound.
(Photograph by Jeff Shultz; reprinted with permission)

10

The Ice Factory

"The ice is like a mean dog, he always waits for you to stop watching
him and then he tries to get you."
— ANTHROPOLOGIST RICHARD K. NELSON,
Hunters of the Northern Ice

ALASKANS CALLED it "the ice factory." Norton Sound, a forbidding inlet of the Bering Sea some 150 miles long and 125
miles across at its widest point, appeared from afar to be an
endless expanse of solid ice that stretched until it met the sky. But the
distant view was deceptive, for the closer you got to the sound, the
more conscious you became that the ice was in a constant state of
change and re-creation. Huge swaths would suddenly break free and
drift out into the sea or a long narrow lead of water would open up
and widen. Depending upon the temperature, wind, and currents, the
ice could assume various configurations—five-foot-high ice hummocks, a stretch of glare ice, or a continuous line of pressure ridges,
which look like a chain of mountains across the sound. Not surprisingly, even among people whose valor on ice had been proved, Norton Sound was considered the most perilous kind of terrain to cross.

Then there was the wind. It was a given that on Norton Sound the
wind howled and that life along these shores would be a constant
struggle against a force that tried to beat you back at every step of
every task. But when the wind blew out of the east, people took special note. These winds were shaped into powerful tunnels, and gusts
barreled down mountain slopes and through river valleys, spilling out

onto the sound at speeds of more than 70 miles per hour. They could flip sleds, hurl a driver off the runners, and drag the wind chill down to minus 100 degrees. Even more terrifying, when the east winds blew, the ice growing out from shore often broke free and was sent out to sea in large floes.

At night, the star-lit hummocks cast deep shadows over a shoreline that already seemed prehistoric with its crags and barren capes, all hardened off with a wind-crusted covering of snow. No campfires or cannery lights twinkled on the horizon, for although there was a rich marine life, the Native villages and white outposts were few and far between. Conditions were simply too harsh and dangerous here; over 380 miles of coastline, the distance from New York to Quebec, there were only six main villages. On the southern shore of the sound stood St. Michael, formerly a Russian fort and fur depot that over the years had become a Native village.[1] Sixty miles or so east of St. Michael was Unalakleet (*YOU-na-la-kleet*—"the place where the east wind blows"), a quiet, industrious village of schooner builders and Native hunters. The village is at the end of the Kaltag portage, the overland route through mountains that linked the Yukon River with the Bering Sea. Nearly forty miles northeast along the coast, before a traveler reached the bulge of Cape Denbigh, was Shaktoolik, the Native village that had become a major center for the wandering commercial

---

1. In 1833, the Russian-American Company built a fort in St. Michael and a storage depot for furs trapped in the Interior awaiting shipment to Russia. After the United States bought the territory, the U.S. Army continued to maintain a fort there. St. Michael had been the commercial and population center for Northwest Alaska as well as a port for goods and passengers heading up the Yukon River looking for gold or furs. The town was eclipsed by Nome when gold was discovered in 1898, and in 1923 it became redundant as a transit point to the Interior when the Alaska Railroad was completed. By 1925, St. Michael had declined to about three hundred people, most of them Eskimo from nearby villages who had been wiped out by a measles epidemic in 1900 and the influenza pandemic in 1918–19. The rusting relics of steamships and gold mining equipment littered St. Michael's beach. By the end of 1925, the U.S. military fort too would be abandoned.

reindeer herds of the northwest.[2] Unalakleet had once been the ter-
minus of the winter Native trade route between Eskimos and
Athabaskans, who first forged the route over the portage, and Shaktoolik was once the southernmost settlement of the Mahlemuit
group. Now, both villages were stops on the mail trail and designated
as the transfer points for the serum en route to Nome.

On the northern coast of Norton Sound the villages were even
smaller, from Koyuk, set in the bend of an inlet a mile up a river, to
the Eskimo Roadhouse at Isaac's Point, and beyond that, Elim, a mission and reindeer reserve. Finally, about ten miles farther west, at
Cape Darby, was six-mile Golovin Bay. From here, there were ninety
more miles of varied, craggy terrain to Nome. A few old mining villages like Bluff, Solomon, and Port Safety dotted the coast, but by
1925 they served mainly as roadhouses for weary travelers.

On Cape Denbigh, at a site called "Iyatayet," twelve miles northeast
of Shaktoolik, archeologists have found traces of early man dating back
eight thousand years. By 1925, the Eskimos in these Norton Sound villages were still keeping to a subsistence lifestyle based on hunting seal
and fish far out on the ice, although with the coming of fur traders,
whalers, and gold miners, the Eskimos along much of the sound were
taking advantage of new tools and techniques the white man had
brought them. In addition, they had improved their livelihood by
freighting supplies by dogsled, herding reindeer, or sculpting figurines
and cribbage boards out of ivory. In return, the Eskimos passed on to the
whites knowledge developed over thousands of years—knowledge that
allowed them to survive winters so close to the Arctic Circle.

At an early age, Eskimo children could already identify every
headland and inlet of the sound and could orient themselves quickly
by reaching down from the sled and feeling blindly for the tiny ice

2. The richness and subtlety of the Eskimo language can be seen just in the
naming of Shaktoolik. The word means "sandbar," after the location of the
town. And it also means "stretched out." One Eskimo in Unalakleet described
yet another meaning: "Further, it means the feeling you have when you have
been going toward a place for so long that it seems that you will never get there."

waves called *sastrugi*, which formed in the same configuration at every freeze and mirrored the topography on shore.

To them, the coast of Norton Sound was a neighborhood, like any other neighborhood. Just as a resident of a European or U.S. city could rattle off the names of stores on streets and know which neighborhoods were safer than others, the Eskimos of Norton Sound could tell you the various conditions of the ice off Isaac's Point (also known as Bald Head) compared to those off Shaktoolik. They paid close attention to the shorefast ice, which grew out from shore every winter. It could vary in length from a few feet, usually around points and capes, to several miles. The relatively stable and safe shorefast ice (no ice should ever be considered totally safe) ended at what was called the flaw edge, or hinge, where it met ice that had formed in place. Beyond the flaw edge, the ice was more dangerous, and under the right conditions of wind and current, it could break up and begin to drift out to sea. It was the first ice to go when the east wind blew onto Norton Sound.

Eskimo children learned how to read the color of ice to tell them whether a particular stretch was safe to cross. Darks spots were signs of thin, unstable ice: the seawater was close beneath. A certain shade of light gray indicated that the ice had built up far enough above the seawater and thus was thick enough for travel. A dog team too could help detect thin ice. It was believed that when dogs suddenly strayed off course, it was because they felt slight changes in moisture on the surface through their paws.

There were times, however, when even an Eskimo made a mistake and realized too late that the ice beneath him was beginning to bend and break. In such a situation, he would not stop moving, as most of us would reflexively be inclined to do, but instead would spread his legs to distribute more widely the support of his weight and then slide forward with both feet on the surface.[3] As a last resort, he would lie

3. According to Richard K. Nelson, this technique may have been learned from watching polar bears, which can walk over ice too thin to support a human by spreading their paws until their bellies nearly touch the surface and then sliding forward (Nelson, *Hunters of the Northern Ice*, 21).

down, stretch out his arms and legs, and shimmy along until he came upon safe ground. This technique had its own dangers in cold weather, because thin ice was moist and would eventually soak a traveler's clothes.

An important tool for ice travel was an unaak, a seven-foot pole with a spike on one end and a hook on the other. With the spike end, an Eskimo hunter could stab as he walked at the snow-covered ice in front of him, gauging its thickness. The hook end was a real survival tool. If he fell through the ice, he could grab onto the edge of the remaining ice, preventing himself from being swept under by the current. If he found himself stranded on a floe but saw a smaller floe closer to the shore, he could use the hook end to pull the smaller floe close enough for him to cross over onto it, using each passing floe as another stepping-stone back to shore.

EARLY SATURDAY morning on January 31, the fourth day of the relay, two men—Myles Gonangnan, a full-blooded Eskimo, and the Norwegian Leonhard Seppala—stood on opposite sides of Norton Sound, unaware of each other's location, and studied the ice and the wind. They each had a decision to make. They could take an over-water route, thereby cutting off a great deal of time, or they could follow an onshore trail that skirted the sound. In either direction, the trail route was safer, and Seppala had already been warned not to attempt an ice crossing. For neither man would the decision be based on courage or even stamina—but solely on which way the wind blew.

Over the past few days, the wind had been blowing onshore, pushing water in from the Bering Sea and raising the level of the sound, which had weakened the ice. But as long as the wind continued to blow from that quarter, there would be little cause for alarm. The ice would continue to break up, as it always does, but it would merely drift toward shore. But sometime during the night, the wind's direction had shifted. It was now blowing offshore, from the northeast, and getting stronger.

A little before five o'clock that morning, Gonangnan had received the serum at Unalakleet from his fellow Eskimo and townsman, Victor Anagick, who had traveled down from the Old Woman shelter cabin on the portage.[4] Leaving it inside Traeger's store to warm near the heat of his iron stove, Gonangnan set out to examine conditions on Norton Sound. A few minutes beyond Unalakleet, he would have to decide whether to take the trail route northeast into the foothills or the shortcut route over the ice. The ice route ran several miles out from shore and under the shadow of Besboro Island, an enormous, uninhabited crag that had long ago broken off from the mainland bluffs.

The shortest route of all would have been to cut straight across the sound, which meant heading northwest in a direct line to Nome. But in the middle of the sound was a large body of open water called a polynya, which was kept free of ice most of the season by a constant eddying. As ice formed in the area of the polynya, wind and current pushed it toward the edge, where it compacted and was then driven into the southerly moving ice pack of the Bering Sea. It made a terrifying grinding noise, like that of giant bulldozers dragging their metal buckets against concrete.

Gonangnan studied the giant field of ice as it creaked and sighed, and by the light of the moon he could see the whole body slightly rise and fall. The sea was rolling in from beneath. Somewhere out in the distance there was open water, spray exploding off whitecaps and floes rumbling and fragmenting. In the cavernous sky above, the stars twinkled with unusual clarity. Behind him, the wind was growing stronger, the gusts more frequent. The signs were clear: a storm was brewing and could well land full force on the coast within twenty-four to forty-eight hours. The question was no longer whether the sea would break up but when. He would not risk taking the shortcut.

Gonangnan returned to the store, picked up the serum, and tied

4. Anagick and a driver known as "Jackscrew" carried the serum over the portage. Jackscrew received the serum from Patsy at Kaltag and then traveled forty miles to Old Woman, where he handed off the serum to Anagick.

the package down in his sled. It was about five-thirty in the morning when he took off for the foothills behind Unalakleet. A few hours later, across the sound, Leonhard Seppala, unaware that the relay had changed, made his decision. He would cross the sound.

FOR THE first twelve miles from Unalakleet, the inland trail ran parallel to the coast, up and down a series of hills with bared slopes and sharp turns, before coming back briefly to shore. The trees along the route offered some shelter but provided little protection from the wind and created their own hazards on the sharp turns.

In the rising wind, Gonangnan headed over the slippery surface of the lagoon behind Unalakleet and then turned inland and climbed steadily up a 300-foot rise into the hills. It was a steep ascent that required alternating between pushing the sled from behind at a jog and pedaling from the runners. Drifts created by the wind and a recent snowfall had built up on the trail and the dogs punched their way through, slowing down in stretches of heavy snow, then speeding up on the stretches of hard-packed trail. But the wind had gotten too much of a head start on Gonangnan. Soon, the trail became too heavily drifted with snow for the dogs. They wallowed in it, unable to get traction. Gonangnan had to stop the team and strap on his snowshoes in preparation for breaking trail.

Breaking trail was a slow and laborious process. A driver had to anchor the sled, take off his own gloves to put on snowshoes, and then jog back and forth over the trail until he had packed down enough snow for the dogs to get through. Whenever there was an easy stretch, he would get back on the sled and ride the runners to catch his breath. A trailbreaker could easily go over a bad stretch of trail three times before the ground was tamped down enough for the dogs. Usually, freighters and mail drivers hired local men to go out ahead and do the job for them to save them time and energy. Gonangnan, of course, had no such luxury.

It took Gonangnan several hours before he finally reached the abandoned fish camp at the point where the trail came back down to the shore. He had been on the trail for about five hours and had managed only twelve miles. It was dismal progress. He built a small fire in one of the abandoned huts and set the serum nearby. He knew the worst was yet to come. The wind outside was blowing harder with each passing hour.

From the fishing camp, the trail ran for five miles up and down over steep ridges until it reached the Blueberry Hills. The Blueberry Hills' summit is 1,000 feet high and the ascent to its exposed ridge top is considered one of the most difficult climbs on the trail to Nome, requiring every ounce of energy from dogs and driver. At the end of the ridge, the trail makes a sharp turn to the west and heads down a steep three-mile descent to the beach for the final stretch to Shaktoolik.

There were several wind tunnels along this route which produced unexpected gusts that hit like body blows. There would be no more abandoned camps or roadhouses for shelter. The only place he might find some relief from the wretched wind would be huddled behind his sled or a boulder, curled up into a ball inside his parka.

If all went well, it would take Gonangnan another nine hours to reach Shaktoolik. The eight dogs on his team were not fast but they were heavily coated and powerful. And they knew the trail. He had traveled hundreds of miles with these dogs along this very coastline, and they were accustomed to gales and heavy loads and the miles of snow and ice that seemed to go on forever.

After warming himself and the serum for about fifteen minutes, Gonangnan headed back out on the trail and began the exhausting climb. For the next several hours he alternated between running behind the sled and riding the runners. The varied terrain required him to be constantly on the move and on the alert. When the wind blows, it shapes the trail, and as a team climbs, the sled skids sideways and downhill. The driver must constantly fight the force of gravity. With knees bent and hands locked tightly to the sled, he pedals vigorously, trying to kick the sled back up into line with the dogs. When on the sled, he hikes out, putting all his weight over the uphill runner to create a little friction. The dogs, too, struggle against the drift of the sled, and the wheel dogs take the brunt. Each time the sled slips downhill, the force nearly jerks the wheel dogs off their feet and they must dig into the snow with their claws to regain footing.

As Gonangnan battled up the summit, the wind came at him nearly head-on, picking up walls of snow and dumping them across the trail. Snow was "blowing so hard," Gonangnan would later recall, "that eddies of drifting, swirling snow passing between the dogs' legs and under the bellies made them appear to be fording a fast running river."

Suddenly, the world closed in on him. It was a whiteout. The horizon ahead had been swallowed up between the overcast sky of the growing storm and the endless white line of the Blueberry Hills. He could not make out the jumbled ice of the sound below. He could not even see it. He was in a world without shade or contour, where every point of visual reference had vanished. It was a northern vertigo, a physical experience unlike any other, where one loses one's sense of balance in the absence of shadows and edges. A dog driver on the trail could no longer tell whether there was a dip or a bump ahead, or whether the dogs had made a wrong turn and were heading off the edge of the ridge.

The team veered sharply to the west and the sled picked up speed. They had begun the descent back to the beach. This section of the trail, although protected from the wind, is notoriously icy and most drivers usually prepare before heading down. They will unhook a few dogs from their tuglines and begin the descent with their foot on the brake, slowing down the sled before dropping off what one musher described as "the edge of the planet." To add friction, some will wrap chains called roughlocks around the runners, and if they have to, they will inch down the slope in stretches of controlled speed, stopping whenever they begin to accelerate too rapidly. Even with these precautions a driver could find himself in trouble.

There would be no such preparation time for Gonangnan. In the whiteout, he did not even realize he had reached the edge until he flew off it like a runaway locomotive. On a steep grade, a sled picks up speed faster than the team and can run right over the wheel dogs. The driver struggles for control of his unwieldy vehicle. He must jam the brake into the icy trail until his leg hurts and at the same time lean into the high side of the trail. The sled bangs into hard drifts and can slide at a right angle to the team. If the runners catch an edge, the sled may flip, tumbling the entire team, the contents of the sled, and the driver hundreds of feet down to the beach.

That day, Gonangnan was lucky. As he neared Norton Sound, the whiteout conditions cleared and he could see the beach below. The sled began to slow down. He had made it safely down the descent. But as he well knew, the final miles once he returned to the shoreline would provide a different yet equally unnerving challenge. Out in the open on the sound there was nothing to block the wind, which shot down the Koyuk River valley and across the sound, slamming into the low-lying spit of Shaktoolik in a noise like thunder. The headwinds can be in excess of 50 mph, the gusts even more. They can polish the trail into slick windows of glare ice, which sparkle the colors of jade and light blue. Dogs struggle for a toehold and drivers fight for every inch of ground.

By 11:00 A.M., the wind was blowing at gale force, about 40 miles per hour. The wind chill was down to at least minus 70 degrees, for the air that feeds the gusts comes down from the Arctic. Gonangnan and his dogs had been traveling for about nine hours now, and it would take him another three or four hours to make it across this stretch of ice. Gonangnan mushed on. The drifting particles of snow and sand hurtled toward him like a white wall. Four grueling hours later, Shaktoolik appeared on the horizon.

It was about 3:00 P.M. when Gonangnan arrived at Shaktoolik, and still there was no sign of Seppala. No one actually knew where Seppala was on the trail. It was possible that he had been delayed or that he had already come across the sound, passed through Shaktoolik without resting, and was now on his way to Unalakleet. Gonangnan, however, had not seen him on the trail.

Mark Summers had prepared for this eventuality, asking Henry Ivanoff, a Russian Eskimo who captained a schooner on the sound in the summers, to be ready to take the serum. Ivanoff sat in the store waiting for the serum to warm while Gonangnan gave him the last few details about the weather outside. While he might not be the ideal man for the job, Ivanoff would do his best. And so he set off along the shore ice of Norton Sound, bound for Ungalik.

THAT SAME Saturday afternoon, Welch and Morgan continued their vigilance. For the past eleven days, they had been monitoring and caring for an increasing number of patients. Today, three more children had come down with the disease, pushing the caseload to twenty-seven. There were thirty suspects and at least eighty people who had come in contact with the bacteria; and now there was no more antitoxin. A new fear had taken hold of Welch. Among his patients was Margaret Curran, whose father ran the roadhouse out at Solomon. Margaret had recently gone out there to help her father cook for guests. Had she spread the disease beyond Nome? Welch was not taking any chances. "Would advise keeping all government nurses at their stations as they are all I have to depend on outside of Nome and it seems inevitable that diphtheria will occur at some of these stations in near future," he wired to the authorities in Washington. "If things get bad may have to establish separate contagious hospital for Natives. . . ."

Mayor Maynard urged people in town to avoid using the telephones to keep the lines clear for emergencies.

A freelance reporter in Nome working for the Universal Service press agency captured the mood in Nome. "Nome Situation Critical; All Hope Rests on Dogs," E. R. Hyldahl wrote in a story that was picked up by the Seattle press. "The situation in diphtheria stricken Nome is extremely critical. . . . There is nothing left to stop the ravages of the disease. Nome is in a state of terrible anxiety while the entire population is waiting for the dogs. All hope is in the dogs and their heroic drivers. . . . Nome appears to be a deserted city. All streets are empty."

Later that same day Welch was given an update on the relay: Gonangnan had left Unalakleet early that morning and all the mushers on the line had been told to keep an eye out for Seppala. With or without Seppala, it was hoped that the serum would reach Nome as early as the next day.

Welch heard the news with relief. In a telegram to the Public Health Service, he wrote: ". . . have received information that 300,000 units antitoxin will arrive tomorrow at noon STOP If you could be here alone you could realize what this means to me STOP."

AROUND THE same time Seppala, too, was feeling confident. Earlier that morning, just a few hours after Gonangnan had set off on the inland route, Seppala had thrown off the cautions of Summers and others and chosen the shortcut across Norton Sound. It was a good move. He had made the crossing.

The wind was behind him now and he was grateful. A storm was clearly brewing and the wind continued to blow hard. The snow was lifting up off the ground in an explosion of hard, fine crystals, but he was moving with the wind so it did not matter much to him. In fact, the tailwind had made for a fast journey. He had just left the fishing camp of Ungalik and now the dogs were speeding toward Shaktoolik over the last twenty-three miles of shorefast ice.

Seppala had covered nearly 170 miles in the past three days and so far he had been lucky with the weather and the ice. Although he could not see the town through the haze of snow, Seppala knew that Shaktoolik was only minutes away. When he reached the roadhouse there, he would decide whether or not to push further down the coast to Unalakleet. To avoid a delay, he wanted to be off the Bering Sea before the storm hit full force. As far as he knew, he still had more than 100 miles to travel before meeting the serum, and he needed to spare himself and the dogs the exhausting ordeal of battling a storm and dangerous ice.

Suddenly, Togo and the dogs picked up speed. They were racing but after what? And then he saw it. There was another sled dog team up ahead. It wasn't moving. Instead, the driver was standing in the middle of the team, flailing his arms. A reindeer had wandered out on the trail and his dogs were fighting to get at it, all snarled up in a tangle of lines and flying fur. Now Seppala's dogs wanted to join the pursuit of game and they put on a burst of speed. Seppala held on tight. It was like being at the end of the line in a game of "crack the whip," which Nome's children played on their ice skates out on the Bering Sea.

When the other driver saw the Siberian Huskies coming toward him, he knew he had more important things to do than get his dogs away from the reindeer. There was only one man who could be out on the trail today with a team of Siberians heading in the opposite direction. He began to wave his arms frantically, determined to catch Seppala's attention.

But Seppala, who could not make out what the driver was shouting above the whistling of the wind, had no intention of stopping to help. He could not afford the delay.

Togo was approaching the team rapidly. Henry Ivanoff made one last attempt. His dogs had probably broken a few harnesses in the fight and some may even have been injured. If he failed to get Seppala's attention, he would have to return to Shaktoolik and take the time to mend the harnesses and find more dogs.

Ivanoff ran toward Seppala as the musher raced past: *"The serum! The serum! I have it here!"*

Seppala at first did not believe what he had heard. He slammed on the sled brake. The brake made little purchase against the snow and it was only after some distance that he managed to stop the dogs and turn them around, into the wind. By the time Seppala made his way back to Ivanoff, the driver had stopped the fight. He ran over to Seppala with the serum and told him of the change of plan. The epidemic had spread rapidly since Seppala left Nome on January 28 and more drivers had been added to the relay in order to speed it up. It was Seppala's job now to carry the serum back across Norton Sound and on to the roadhouse at Golovin, where Charlie Olson was waiting for the handoff.

Alarmed by the news, Seppala started off at once for Ungalik, the fishing camp twenty-three miles to the north. He had to decide what to do. The route back across Norton Sound had become much more dangerous since this morning. The wind was building and it was beginning to get dark, so he would not be able to see or hear the ice. He could take the long route around the shore, but neither he nor Nome could afford the extra day of travel. Seppala had his own daughter to worry about. Sigrid was only eight years old, his only child, and he had no way of knowing if she was on Dr. Welch's growing list.

Seppala may have had his doubts about recrossing Norton Sound that afternoon, but the rest of the world did not. In the lower 48 that same Saturday afternoon, former residents of Nome were regaling the press with tales of the courageous musher who would save the town. No one back in the states could even assure the press that Seppala would meet up with the relay, given the change of plans. But none of that mattered. Most of those talking were former sourdoughs, who had moved to the states several years ago, but who still had the gambling spirit of the gold rush days in them and were "ready to bet their final ounce of dust" that Seppala would reach his destination in record time.

"There is no man in Alaska better fitted to undergo the great hazard than he," Esther Darling, who used to work with the musher Scotty Allan, told the *Berkeley Gazette*. "Only a man of long experience on the trail dares to take a trip such as that Seppala has undertaken when the thermometer goes to 58 below. The slightest misstep will result in death. The danger is that a man usually does not realize he is freezing until his brain becomes numb. Then he goes crazy and that, of course, is the end."

Bob Lilly, who once drove with Seppala, chimed in from his home in San Francisco: Seppala "always argued that there's nothing—animals, airplanes, automobiles—that can beat the dog for transportation in Alaska. He's going to prove it or they'll pick him up frozen in death. This race means everything to Seppala. For years he has trained his dogs with the belief that they are the only sure source of the North. . . . When Nome called for aid, and men measured the route . . . the airplane was unsafe, and the package that meant life to Nome was entrusted to the sled dogs—Seppala's sled dogs."

"There isn't any quit in him," said a former mayor of Nome,

George Baldwin. "There isn't any quit to any of those chaps, for that matter—Kaasen, Wild Bill Shannon—he's an Irishman—Edgar Kallands or any of 'em. Those dogs of theirs will get them there quick."

The kind of confidence these Alaskan sourdoughs had in Seppala, Seppala had in his lead dog, Togo. When he saw the huts of Ungalik up ahead, Seppala turned left without hesitation and headed out across Norton Sound. It was now dark. The temperature, as he would later estimate, was minus 30 degrees and the gale was in his face. With the wind chill, it was a brutal 85 below. There was nothing Seppala could do but drive as if he were in a race.

Seppala had been out on the sound with Togo once before in a northeast gale. He had been just a few miles offshore when, in a lull between gusts, he heard an ominous crack. He ordered Togo to "haw," but the leader had already felt the crack and was heading at top speed toward the nearest point on land. He was closing in to shore when Togo inexplicably reared up and somersaulted back onto his teammates. Seppala shouted angrily. This was no time for circus stunts. He ran up to Togo to see what was the matter and as he neared the dog, he saw why he had stopped. No more than six feet ahead was an open channel of water. The lead was growing wider before Seppala's eyes. He was on a floe, drifting out toward the sea. He straightened out the dogs and skirted the edges of the floe, looking for an opportunity to escape, but there was none. It had been noon when he set out from shore at Isaac's Point and now night was falling and the temperature dropping. There was nothing he could do but curl up with his dogs, conserve his strength and his warmth, and hope for a shift in the wind to bring him in to shore.

Several hours later, no such shift had occurred and Seppala's anguish grew. His dogs sensed the change in his mood and let out a long and low plaintive cry. Then Togo gave a short yelp.

The leader had sensed a shift: the wind was beginning to blow onshore. Seppala hitched his team back up and waited. He drifted for nine more hours until he could see the shoreline only a few hundred yards ahead. The ice raft was closing in on a floe that had jammed up against the shorefast ice. Seppala mushed along the perimeter to find a place to jump off. The closest point on the raft to the floe was about five feet—too wide for Seppala to jump. But if he could get Togo to the other side, the dog could pull the two floes together. Seppala tied a long towline to Togo's harness, picked him up, and hurled him across the open channel. Most dogs would have run away after a stunt like that, but as Seppala later reported, "Togo seemed to understand what he had to do." Once on the other side, Togo dug his nails into the floe and lurched toward shore. The line snapped. Togo spun around and looked back across the chasm at Seppala. The line slipped into the water. Seppala was speechless. He had just been given a death sentence.

Animal psychologists have a phrase for the ability to find solutions. It is called "adaptive intelligence." The icy lead separating Togo from Seppala was keeping the dog from his reward: reuniting with his master and his team. Togo had been born and bred a northern sled dog and it was part of his instinct now to pull. From an early age he had been exposed to an amazing array of daily challenges that had improved his ability to learn and in some cases to solve problems. He had traveled over various terrain in summer and winter and had spent most of his entire day for the past twelve years watching and working with Seppala as the team traveled out in the gold fields and to towns across Alaska.

As Seppala stood staring across the lead at Togo, the dog dove into the water, snapped the line up into his mouth, and struggled back out onto the jammed-up floe. Holding the line tightly in his jaws, Togo rolled over the line "until it was twice looped about his shoulders" and began to pull. The floe started to move and Togo continued to pull until it was close enough for Seppala and his teammates to jump safely across.

Now, as Seppala and Togo crossed Norton Sound in the late afternoon of Saturday, January 31, Seppala had no choice but to put his faith in Togo one more time. It would be the last time the two would cross the sound together. As Seppala feared, it was already too dark for his own eyes to see anything. The wind was deafening. Occasionally, he leaned out over the sled listening for any clue that the ice was cracking up. The sound was holding, and Togo seemed unfazed by the wind, covering the miles of trail with his head held low and his body level in deep concentration. He kept a straight course, despite the hummocks and slippery patches of ice that loomed up in his path.

At 8:00 P.M. that evening, Seppala and Togo pulled up the bank at Isaac's Point on the other side of Norton Sound. The dogs had traveled an incredible eighty-four miles that day, half of it against the wind, and they were all worn out. Togo and the team had averaged eight miles per hour. They were hungry and needed a rest before battling the wind for the next fifty miles to Golovin. Seppala unhooked the dogs and fed them salmon and seal blubber. They wasted no time in curling up their tails and going to sleep.

With the dogs cared for, Seppala drew his sled into the roadhouse and unlashed the package. He undid the wrappings of fur and canvas down to the paper cartons enclosing the serum. From the appearance of the cartons, Seppala was certain that the serum inside had frozen, so he placed it as close to the fire as he dared. While the serum warmed, Seppala slid into his reindeer sleeping bag and took a few hours of rest. At this point, he could only hope.

Outside, the wind roared down the peninsula and out onto Norton Sound, where the ice exploded in rifle-crack reports. The low-pressure system, which had moved up from the Gulf of Alaska, had arrived. By the following day it would reach its height, unleashing storm-force winds of at least 65 miles per hour as the mushers made the final dash to Nome.

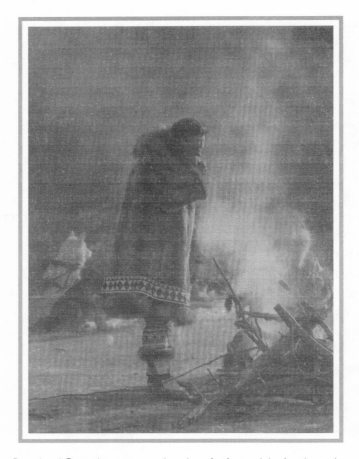

Leonhard Seppala camps on the edge of a frozen lake for the night.
(Photograph courtesy of Bill Hanks and Sigrid Seppala-Hanks)

11

Cold Glory

"There are only three things that a Northern dog is really afraid of: a blizzard, thin ice and the cracking sound of ice on a cold day."
— SCOTTY ALLAN

A T 2:00 A.M. on Sunday, February 1, the fifth day of the relay, Nichuk, the owner of the roadhouse at Isaac's Point, shook Seppala awake. The storm that had been heading up from the south over the past two days had arrived, and it was time for Seppala to leave. Removing the serum package from its spot near the stove, Seppala wrapped it inside his sleeping bag, covered it with a sealskin robe, and tied it down with a blanket in his sled. As an extra precaution, he covered it with additional animal skins. With a storm like this, he was taking no chances. He pushed the sled out the door.

The wind was howling and the ice on Norton Sound hissed and cracked. While Seppala harnessed the last dogs to the gang line, an old Eskimo emerged from the roadhouse and headed toward him.

"Maybe you go more closer shore," he said quietly. Eskimos did not take unnecessary chances on the trail and this time even Seppala understood that he had to be cautious.

Much of the trail between Isaac's Point and Golovin, where according to the new plan Seppala would hand the serum off to Charlie Olson, was a few miles offshore, bypassing a number of craggy points that jutted out from the coast. Although the trail would be rougher, Seppala decided to stay within a few hundred feet of the land.

It was about minus 40 below now and as he edged down the bank at Isaac's Point he could feel the wind building in strength. The Eskimo had been right: this was no time to be out over water. The ice he had crossed a day earlier had already broken up and around him he saw cakes of ice threatening to come loose. The cracks seemed to be getting closer, and in some places open water was just a few feet away. Water spurted up through cracks and the ice heaved. Togo zigzagged around the weak spots and several times put on a burst of speed toward shore. At times, blizzard conditions obscured Seppala's vision. Once the last bay had been crossed, the team turned toward the mainland, putting the ice floes behind them, and Seppala breathed a little easier.

A few hours later, the entire section of ice over which they had come broke up in chunks and blew out to sea.

Once firmly on shore, Seppala stopped the team and rubbed the dogs down, brushing off a layer of ice and snow that had formed over their faces, drying off their paws, and tending to any cuts on their feet. Although the most dangerous part of the run was behind them, the most physically challenging part was just starting. They would have to climb a series of ridges to the 1,200-foot summit of Little McKinley, which overlooks Golovin Bay.

Many mushers consider that climb to be the toughest part of the trail to Nome. The exposed ridges stretch out over eight miles. The downgrades are steep and the dogs and drivers have little time to recover from one ridge before they have to breathe in deep and charge up the next. By the time the summit of Little McKinley is reached, the teams have climbed about 5,000 feet. Seppala's dogs were being asked to make the climb with less than five hours of rest, and after they had traveled for four and a half days and covered 260 miles of trail. With few reserves to call on, the team began to stumble from exhaustion. But they did not stop, and strained up the final ascent, then raced three miles down to Dexter's roadhouse in Golovin.

Some thirteen hours after the start at Isaac's Point, Seppala's team arrived at its destination and passed the serum to Charlie Olson. It had been a seamless effort. Since Seppala had picked up the serum from Ivanoff on the shore ice of Norton Sound, he and his dogs had traveled 135 miles, more than two and a half times the distance covered by any of the other drivers. And this was done at top speed, in blizzard conditions over heaving ice. He and the dogs had survived the ruthless challenge of Norton Sound and saved at least a day off the critical time schedule. Looking at them, you would never know. All they needed was a rest. It was a testament to Seppala's training, condtioning, and skills on the trail.

The time was a little before 3:00 P.M. Now, all that stood between Golovin and Nome was the final stretch of seventy-eight miles.

THE STORM was making itself felt beyond Golovin. On the same day, a Sunday, Nome awoke to the sound of the wind rising. It had been nearly two weeks since Billy Barnett's death. The streets were empty; not a single parishioner was headed up to Sunday mass and there were no children skating out on the Snake River. Earlier in the week, some boys had been allowed out to throw snowballs at each other, albeit at a safe distance. Now even they had retreated to the safety of their cabins. Loose boards began to rattle, and snow pellets blew against the walls with a *pock, pock* sound that grew in volume and intensity.

Out on the Sandspit, Nurse Morgan struggled against the wind, visiting as many families as possible before her vision became obscured by the blowing snow and the cold became unbearable. Since the death of Bessie Stanley, the first Eskimo to die from diphtheria, the Sandspit had been under a strict lockdown enforced by teachers from the government-run Native School. They patrolled the streets to make sure the quarantine was obeyed and that every household had enough food, coal, and water to last through the storm.

Across town, Dr. Welch went through the medical reports, visited patients, and did what he could to keep up with the number of victims. Another case had been identified and Welch made a frightening observation. There were twenty-eight cases in Nome now, and "even if the dogs manage to arrive with the supply there will be sufficient antitoxin to care for only 30 people." He told this to the local United Press reporter Robert McDowell, who was unaware at the time that he, his wife, and infant daughter would soon be added to the list of the ill.

As dire as that sounded, the more serious concern was that the drivers would never make it to Nome. This was already shaping up as an extraordinary blizzard. Even experienced mushers wouldn't want to tempt fate under these conditions. If just one driver in the relay got lost or blown off course by the storm and could not reach the warmth of a roadhouse, the ampoules of serum would eventually freeze, expand, and crack, thus ruining the supply.

Caught between the need for serum and the possibility that a heroic attempt to mush through the storm could result in the loss of the first shipment, Curtis Welch decided to call a meeting of the Board of Health and ask them to stop the relay. The loss of a few hours or even a few days, he explained, was not as important as the safety of the shipment. Twenty-eight lives were now depending on the antitoxin reaching Nome intact. The health board members agreed.

In an attempt to reach the mushers, Mayor Maynard picked up the phone and requested the operator to put him through to Pete Curran, the roadhouse keeper at Solomon. Maynard told Curran that when Gunnar Kaasen arrived from Bluff with the serum, he should be ordered to remain in Solomon until the storm abated and it was safe to resume travel. A call was also sent out to Port Safety, where Ed Rohn, the last driver in the relay, was informed that the rescue attempt had been temporarily halted.

No one in the room knew if these calls would have any effect: the exact location of the serum was unknown. Because the telephone lines from Nome reached only as far as Solomon and there was no Signal Corps connection with the coast, the last update had been Gonangnan's departure from Unalakleet yesterday morning. It was not even clear whether Gonangnan had met up with Seppala and if Seppala had safely crossed Norton Sound and passed the serum on to Charlie Olson, who was to pass it to Gunnar Kaasen. Kaasen was the penultimate driver in the relay, and he was expected to check in at Solomon before going on to Port Safety.

Still, everyone agreed that putting in the calls had been the right thing to do. Having achieved his goal, Welch walked out into what had become a severe blizzard and made his way over to the Signal Corps station. He had to update Washington on the storm before he too took cover from the winds.

"Violent blizzard now on is delaying progress," he wired his colleagues at the Public Health Service. "Have ordered antitoxin stopped as I wish to take no chances on its freezing or being lost to save a few hours." In a switch from his usual matter-of-fact tone, Welch continued: "Deeply grateful your wire. [A reference to the message Welch had received the day before in which his superiors professed their confidence in his ability to handle the epidemic.] A touch of the human heartens a man. Will try to prove that your confidence is not misplaced."

Out at Port Safety, twenty-one miles from Nome, Rohn received the telephone call from Nome. He could not have agreed more with the decision of the health board. From the window of the roadhouse, he could see the ice beyond the lagoon that separated Port Safety from the Bering Sea. It was, as he described it, in "constant motion from a heavy groundswell." Rohn unhooked the dogs, fed them, and put the sled away. Before settling in for a long rest, he telephoned Nome with a message: the wind was blowing 80 miles per hour, "whirling the snow so that it was impossible for man or beast to face the storm. . . ." As the message came through, the connection crackled and the line went dead. Nome lost what little communication it had with the drivers and it could only pray that the message had reached Kaasen.

It would not.

FIFTY MILES east, on the other side of Cape Nome, Gunnar Kaasen sat in the roadhouse at Bluff. He had no inkling of the meeting in Nome or the decision to hold off the relay. Bluff was a tiny mining village of fewer than forty people, named after the surrounding gray bluffs that towered over the coast. It was situated well east of the telephone lines to Nome.

Kaasen had arrived at the roadhouse sixteen hours earlier, and at five o'clock on Sunday evening he was still sitting by the glowing iron stove, alert for any sounds indicating Olson's arrival. He occasionally opened the door and looked down the trail into the swirling snow.

All Kaasen could hear was the wind as it moaned through the buildings abandoned after the gold rush. It had been years since he could remember such a strong wind, and for a moment he worried that Olson had been pinned down by the storm somewhere out on the trail. He had no way of knowing when or if Olson would arrive, and so he had to stay ready to move out at any moment.

The dogs needed to be fed. There were thirteen of them staked outside in line. Kaasen struggled out the door and fed each one of them salmon and a chunk of tallow. This would provide the necessary calories to keep the dogs warm.

Kaasen had taken a chance in choosing Balto as his lead dog. Named by Seppala after a Laplander who had accompanied the explorer Fridtjof Nansen on his 1888–89 expedition to Greenland, Balto was relatively inexperienced. Seppala considered the animal to be second rate. He was too slow to make the first string, and was used principally to haul freight on short runs.

Kaasen thought more highly of Balto. The dog may not have been as fast as the others, but he was steady and strong.

By 1925, Kaasen and Seppala had already been working together for years organizing Hammon Consolidated's water irrigation system of the gold fields. Kaasen often used the dogs for company and personal trips. The two men came from the same region of Norway, but they could not have been more different. Kaasen was a towering and tough man, six feet two, gruff and introverted. He had a quiet, no-nonsense way about him.

"Either you listened to him or you got thumped on the head," one of his relatives said fondly. Fondly, because the driver had a gentle side, which came out more in acts of kindness than in words. He had a passion for vanilla ice cream and loved to share it with anyone who had an appetite, and he kept the door open to any boy or girl hungry for his wife's famous cinnamon rolls.

Two hours later, around 7:00 P.M., Kaasen heard a faint shout outside. It had to be Olson. Kaasen pushed open the door. It was clear that Olson had had a bitter ride. His hands were too numb from frostbite to unlash the serum, and his seven dogs, short-haired for sled dogs, were stiff in the groin. Kaasen helped the musher inside the roadhouse and sat him down. Then he went back outside to retrieve the serum and bring the team inside. Olson had tied rabbit-fur blankets around each dog's groin, but this was not enough protection. All seven limped into the cabin and lay down stiffly on the floor. "They couldn't have gone much further," Kaasen observed.

It had taken Olson nearly four and a half hours to travel the twenty-five miles from Golovin to Bluff. Putting on the dog blankets had nearly cost him his fingers. The wind chill temperature had been well below minus 70 degrees and in such weather a driver could expose his hands for only minutes at a time before the flesh freezes. It had taken Olson of course much longer to blanket his seven dogs. In the warm cabin, Olson pulled off his gloves. His fingers were white and hard as stone; at best it would be days before their full use would be restored.

As they sat in the roadhouse, Olson told his story.

The wind had repeatedly blown the team off the trail and at the lagoon just outside Golovin a gust of hurricane force slammed into the rig, hurling him and the team into a nearby drift. Olson had fought in the dark to dig his way out and untangle the dogs, but the struggle had worn him out. Despite his two parkas and a double fur hood, the forty-six-year-old bachelor could not keep warm in the blizzard. Olson was as tough as they come in Alaska, accustomed to the rugged demands of mining alone in the northwest. He had seen the worst that the Seward Peninsula could throw at a dog team and for a moment he thought that he would not make it.

Now, looking out the cabin window, Olson could see a vortex of snow in the air. He warned Kaasen to hold off. However much Nome needed the serum, this was not the weather to travel in. Kaasen looked around the room: Olson's fingers were burning with pain; the dogs lay crippled, ragged and exhausted on the floor. It was good advice. Kaasen would heed it, but only to a point.

Two hours later, the wind still had not died down. If anything, it had risen and it was getting colder. It was ten o'clock and the temperature was minus 28, without the wind chill. Snow was coming down fast and being blown by the wind. If he didn't leave now, the trail to Port Safety, thirty-four miles away, would be impassable with drifts. Kaasen stepped outside. In all his twenty-four years in Nome, he had never felt such a blast. One report put the wind's speed in excess of 70 mph. "I had seal mukluks on my feet. They go up to the hips. And I had sealskin pants over them. On my head I had a reindeer parka and hood and a drill parka over that. But the wind was so strong that it went right through the skins."

Kaasen made his decision. "There wasn't any use in waiting." He would head out.

When all thirteen dogs were hooked up to the gang line, he went back inside and got the serum. With his heavy parka reaching below his waist and his face hidden deep inside the fur ruff of his hood, Kaasen loomed in the doorway like some mythological giant of the north. He said a brief good-bye to Olson, opened the door, and stepped back out into the night.

Few drivers had the courage, the know-how, and the dogs to face a blizzard head-on. No amount of movement can keep a musher warm in such conditions. Most travelers caught out in a blizzard stop and make camp. Yet even that can be a dangerous business, for on this coast there are few trees to fuel a fire. A driver has only the sled to hide behind and his sleeping bag, fur robes, and dogs to help keep him warm. He can remain holed up like that for days until the blizzard abates and it is safe to carry on. Sourdoughs had a saying for the times when they found themselves stranded by a blizzard. "We are up against it. Up against it good and strong."

Stumbling through a blizzard, "you don't know whether to pray, curse or cry. You generally do all three together," the All Alaska Sweepstakes racer Scotty Allan once said. "But after a while the blizzard becomes a hated thing with a personality. You get that back to the wall feeling, and like a man in the heat of battle, you forget to feel afraid. You grow to glory in the fight with the damned thing."

A blizzard attacks a musher by causing confusion. His eyelashes freeze shut, his face is pounded by snowy blasts every way he turns, and he loses his sense of direction. "You can't see it. You can't lay hands on it. You can only feel it," Allan said. The stories of the men and dogs who had survived the Alaskan blizzards would pass into legend. Allan once claimed that nine out of ten dogs would turn tail in the face of a blizzard. The fearless ones were prized throughout the Seward Peninsula and these brave few could inspire an entire team. These were the leaders the mushers depended upon for their lives.

Allan left behind a vivid description of mushing in a blizzard. On the final ninety-mile stretch to Nome during the sweepstakes, his team was enveloped in "air thick as smoke with whirling snow. Gritty as salt it was, and stinging like splinters of steel. It baked into my furs and into the coats of my dogs, until we were encased in snow crusts solid as ice. The din deafened me. I couldn't hear, couldn't see, couldn't breathe. I felt as if the dogs and I were fighting all the devilish elements in the universe." Every fifteen minutes, Allan stopped his team and crawled up the gang line, putting a hand on each dog to check his condition. The younger dogs were whining and trying to bury themselves beneath the snow, but every time Allan reached the front of the team, he found the leader, Baldy, "sturdy and brave as a little polar bear . . . a small brave bit of life in that vast, storm-swept waste. . . . I'd melt the ice away from his face and hug him," and then fumble back to the sled. "I was so darned proud and happy over that pup I just couldn't find the words to tell him what I thought of him," Allan said. Kaasen too would have trouble finding the words to describe the courage of his own leader, Balto.

Five miles into the run, Kaasen's worst fears materialized. Since leaving the roadhouse, the wind had sanded the trail down to a hard and fast crust, but here by a ridge a towering drift had formed, blocking the trail. Balto tried to run his way through, but he and the other dogs quickly became mired in the snow. Kaasen waded in after them to clear a path, but he too floundered as the snow rose up to his chest. There was no way the team could get through to the other side except by retreating and then going around the ridge. Kaasen had to turn the dogs around. He grabbed Balto's harness and together they dragged the team in a tight arc through the drift and back out the way they had come. Getting around the ridge would be difficult. Balto had worked largely on the trails to the various dredge sites beyond Nome, and Kaasen was asking the dog to find an unfamiliar trail in unfamiliar territory in the pitch dark of the blizzard. Kaasen could barely see 100 feet ahead of him. Balto lurched forward and tentatively plowed his way through the snow along the back of the ridge. He understood that he had to regain the trail, to find the faint scent of dogs that had pattered before him that winter. Balto kept his nose low to ground, his ears flattened against his head to keep out the wind, as he moved slowly over the snow.

A dog's sense of smell is at least 600 to 700 times more powerful than that of a human and Balto was capable of smelling the tracks left behind by other dogs several feet beneath the snow. A canine's paws too are sensitive and would help Balto feel the hard-packed surface of a trail that had been covered over by new snow. Minutes passed like hours. They were beyond the ridge and still Balto searched. Suddenly, the dog lifted his head and broke out into a run. They were back on the trail.

A few miles farther on, the trail turned hard again as Kaasen entered a valley. It was Topkok River, its frozen surface wiped clean of snow by the wind. His right cheek began to sting with frostbite. Crossing the river, as he neared the west bank, Balto stopped. Kaasen went to the head of the team and saw a large stretch of overflow that Balto had run right into and now refused to go further. It was shallow but deep enough to have soaked the dog's feet. Kassen turned the team off the river, dried Balto's feet, and then moved on.

With the overflow behind them, the team charged over a series of ridges that ran perpendicular to the shore. Each dropped sharply down to a creek and Kaasen found a momentary reprieve from the wind. The last and highest of the ridges was Topkok Mountain, the brutal 600-foot climb with a long, exposed summit. Mushers generally tackled Topkok only in the daylight. The trail hugged the rocky cliffs, but with the wind howling down the slope, a driver could quickly become disoriented. You work your way too far to the south, and you sail off the edge to the beach below. It was here that Seppala nearly lost his life during his first sweepstakes race in 1914. As Kaasen approached the base of Topkok, he stopped for a few minutes, caught his breath, and then, pushing from behind, he urged the dogs on as he charged up the mountain. It seemed that for every step they took forward, the storm pushed them back two. The dogs crawled on their bellies as they fought their way up. Kaasen's right cheek went numb from the cold. "Topkok is hell when it's storming," Kaasen would later recall. "It was storming some when I got up there."

Upon reaching the summit, Kaasen jumped back onto the sled and held on as the dogs raced along the summit. He strained his eyes in the darkness to make sure the dogs were not heading toward the edge. If it had been daytime and calm, Kaasen would have been able to see clear across the coast to Cape Nome, but it was well after midnight now and the storm continued to rage. At the end of the ridge, the team picked up speed and began to race down the far slope of Topkok. They were on the six-mile stretch of flats after Topkok, and the wind was coming across the sloughs and lagoons, picking up snow in such thick veils that Kaasen could barely see his hand in front of his face. His wheel dogs were completely obscured. This stretch of the coast was famous for violent local winds. A series of wind tunnels lines the coast, generating hurricane-force gusts and areas of calm as if someone were flipping off and on a switch. As the team fanned along the curve of the beach, the winds harassed them from the right. This is a dangerous part of the trail, for it ran just behind the dune line, crossing slippery lagoons and bare spots. To the left, on the other side of the line, was sea ice, and open water often lay just a quarter mile offshore. A team can easily drift over the line in a strong wind, and any team that found itself on ice had to turn directly into the wind and fight its way back to the beach.

For more than an hour, the blowing snow had been so thick that Kaasen could not see the trail and could only guess at his position each time Balto crossed another lagoon or creek. He had given control of the team over to Balto and his job now was to hold on. "I didn't know where I was," Kaasen would later recall. "I couldn't even guess." Then, in a lull between gusts, Kaasen recognized a vast depression in the land up ahead as the Bonanza Slough. He was well beyond Solomon. It was two miles back. He had missed the roadhouse, which was just north of the trail. It was then that he made a decision, the most controversial of the entire race. He would push on to Port Safety. He could rest later. It would be a decision he would soon regret.

It was about ten more miles to Port Safety, where Ed Rohn was to take the serum into Nome. As Kaasen headed over across Bonanza Slough, he entered a long blowhole and the wind hit him. It takes a 60- to 70-mph wind to flip a sled, and throughout his journey Kaasen had struggled to keep the rig down. Finally, he was overwhelmed. Entering the blowhole, Kaasen did not have enough strength or weight to keep the sled upright. Several times the sled was hurled off the trail, dragging the dogs with it. Each time, Kaasen had to take off his gloves, untangle the team, and right the sled.

Before crossing to the other side, a final gust slammed into the sled. Kaasen found himself buried in a drift. He crawled in the darkness back to the sled, righted it, and fumbled with the dogs' harnesses. He patted the sled down with his hands to make sure the serum was still in place. He worked his hands up and down the basket, first methodically and then frantically. It was gone. His stomach tightened. The worst had happened. Kaasen dropped to the ground and crawled around the snow, probing in the darkness with his bare hands for the serum. His right hand hit against something hard. He grabbed it. It was the serum. He lashed it back to the sled, gave it a few extra turns with the rope, and fled this devilish stretch of land.

The gust that flipped Kaasen's sled marked a turn in the musher's luck. At the end of the slough, the trail curved to the southwest and the wind was now at his back. In his own words, the going was better and "boosted" him along over the last few miles to the Port Safety roadhouse in a little over an hour.

When he arrived, it was about three o'clock in the morning and the roadhouse was dark. After sending the storm warning to Nome earlier that evening, Ed Rohn had gone to sleep, assuming that Kaasen too would be waiting at Solomon for the storm to abate before heading on to Port Safety.

Kaasen stared up at the roadhouse from the trail. He contemplated waking Rohn. But it would take time for the driver to harness and hitch up his dogs. The wind appeared to be easing, and although he and his dogs were cold, they were still moving fast down the trail. He figured he would make better time if he continued on to Nome.

For the last twenty miles, the trail ran along the beach. The wind continued to die down, but travel was slow and difficult because of heavy drifts. Although his fingers ached with frostbite and several of his dogs were stiffening up, Kaasen was grateful at least to be able to see the path ahead.

Around 5:30 A.M. on Monday, February 2, Kaasen could make out the outline of the cross above St. Joseph's Church. Within a few minutes he pulled up onto Front Street and stopped, exhausted, his eyes stinging from the cold, dry air, outside the door of the Miners & Merchants Bank of Nome.

Witnesses to this drama said they saw Kaasen stagger off the sled and stumble up to Balto, where he collapsed, muttering: "Damn fine dog."

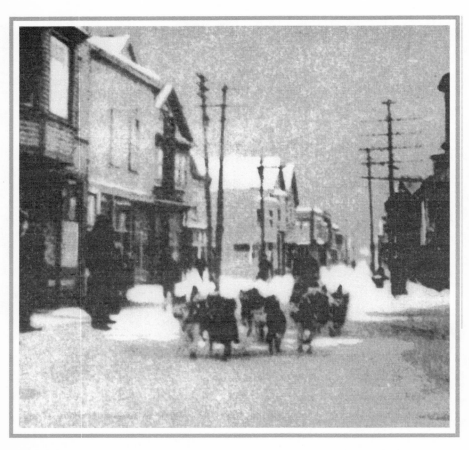

Gunnar Kaasen with Balto in the lead driving down Front Street on February 2, 1925. This was a reenactment of their arrival earlier that morning, staged for photographers. (Authors' collection)

12

Saved!

"Final Dash Brings Antitoxin to Nome, But It Is Frozen. Believe Serum Still Good."

— *The New York Times*, FEBRUARY 3, 1925

THAT MONDAY, February 2, within minutes of Kaasen's arrival, Welch began to unwrap the package. The serum was frozen solid but the vials did not appear to be broken, a testament to the care Dr. Beeson in Anchorage had taken in packing them, as well as the care with which the mushers handled their cargo.[1] The serum would have to be thawed before it could be used, and that would take time. Welch took it to the hospital and put it in a warm room (by Alaskan standards), at 46 degrees. By nine o'clock, the serum in the vials had been partially liquefied and not a single bottle was broken. By 11:00 A.M., the serum was clear and was ready for use.

News of the serum's arrival had spread through town, and the first order of business was to treat the most severe cases. Welch went first to the Winters and McDowell households. John Winters's wife was very ill; she had contracted the disease from her young daughter two days earlier, on January 31, and her condition had deteriorated over the past few hours. Now her husband had come down with the disease.

Robert McDowell, the United Press reporter, had also developed

---

1. According to telegrams sent after the serum's arrival, Dr. Beeson in Anchorage had apparently counteracted any expansion of the serum by using rubber and cork stoppers on each ampoule.

symptoms. His throat was red and swollen and the doctor could see the beginnings of a membrane, so he gave McDowell an initial shot of 5,000 units. The newsman's reports had played an important role in getting the Nome story out to papers across the globe. But now, with his twenty-four-year-old wife and infant daughter under quarantine and suspected of having been infected, he had become the story.

Nurse Morgan, meanwhile, headed over to the Sandspit to give each member of the Stanley family several thousand units of anti-toxin. She went on to visit several other families and immunized each of them.

By early afternoon, more than 10 percent of the 300,000 units had been used up. Many of the same patients would receive a second round of injections, and later that evening several thousand more units of serum were gone. The 300,000 units would be exhausted long before the arrival of the second shipment of 1.1 million units.

Of all the cases that had developed since the start of the relay, Margaret Curran's was the one that frightened Curtis Welch the most. She had developed symptoms earlier in the week, several days after her return to town from her father's roadhouse in Solomon. The implications had weighed heavily on Welch in the final days of the relay. If she had indeed contracted diphtheria, then every traveler who passed through the roadhouse would also have been exposed to the disease. It could be a matter of days before reports of new infections would begin to come in from communities along the coast. The 1.1 million units en route to the ice-free port of Seward had to reach Nome a lot faster than officials had planned.

The shipment had left Seattle by ship on Saturday and it still had to travel by rail from Seward to Nenana before the regular mail could take it to Nome by dogsled. The medicine was expected to arrive in Nenana around the 8th, in six days. The regular mail route journey from Nenana to Nome typically took about twenty-five days.

Time was not on Nome's side, especially if Welch's worst fears about the Curran case turned out to be justified.

At a meeting of the Board of Health that Monday, Welch took a position he had not taken before. It was time, he conceded, to risk all and try to deliver at least half of the next shipment of serum by air, a dangerous gamble. "I should feel much safer if I knew that I would get additional shipment not more than ten days from date," Welch wrote in a telegram that was read by Surgeon General Cumming.

As news of Welch's plight spread, it seemed that many officials now were in agreement that half the shipment should be diverted further up the railroad to Fairbanks, where a plane would be waiting to carry it to Nome.

Everyone, except Governor Bone.

With Welch's assent, Mayor Maynard brought Thompson and Sutherland up to date on the situation. Thompson must have gone right to work on it, for the following day Roy Darling and Ralph Mackie were in the cockpit of the biplane, taking it for a test drive down the main street of Fairbanks in minus-14-degree weather beneath clear skies.

The test run was proof enough to everyone in town that both plane and fliers could take off at a moment's notice. Volunteers began to pack the aircraft with supplies. The excitement was growing in Fairbanks, and in Nome, Welch and the others heard the news with relief.

There was even greater cause for relief when news spread that the 300,000 units that had been brought by dogsled relay seemed to be working. The repeated thawing and freezing did not seem to have damaged the serum's efficacy, and on February 3 it looked as if even those who were seriously ill would recover.

The members of the Winters family were improving and Robert McDowell was on the mend just hours after receiving the medicine.

"I'm carrying on," McDowell said in a dispatch to his colleagues in San Francisco. "My case is not considered serious."

The reporter had to dictate the message to a friend because he was still under quarantine.

But it was not all good news. Later that afternoon, Robert McDowell's daughter developed a grayish white spot in her throat, and his wife, Vera, also appeared to be ill. (Her name does not appear on the medical list of diphtheria patients.) At seven o'clock that evening, Vera drew her final breath, apparently the sixth victim of the epidemic.

Vera McDowell was a prominent woman in Nome. She was the first white girl to be born during the gold rush days, delivered on March 16, 1900, and her loss was felt by many of the townsfolk. Some newspapers attributed her death to diphtheria, but Nome's death records stated the cause as venous air embolism and miscarriage. (Vera was four to five months pregnant.) An air embolism is an infrequent complication of pregnancy, and since she had no symptoms of a sore throat, Vera McDowell probably did not have diphtheria.

But in the chaos of the epidemic, Vera's death was reported across the states, and officials in Washington and the public at large shuddered at the news. The *San Francisco Chronicle*'s headline read: "Six Dead As Plague Gains Added Force."

On Friday, February 6, Vera's parents and close friends got permission to hold a private funeral and led a small procession by horse-drawn hearse to the Belmont Point Cemetery, where the body was placed in a vault until proper burial could be made after the ground had thawed in the spring.

"She was known to every sourdough, miner and prospector in the early days on the Seward Peninsula," McDowell wrote in a terse obituary for the *Seattle Star*.

By Friday afternoon, about one third of the serum had been used. Mayor Maynard, Hammon executive Mark Summers, and "Wrong Font" Thompson again bombarded Bone with messages demanding that he authorize an air flight from Fairbanks.

"If this rate continues you can see how long this shipment will last," Summers said in his telegram.

Bone acknowledged their concern but held his ground. Was it mere stubbornness that precluded him from dividing up the serum, allowing the pilots to make their daring rescue flight? Did Juneau and Washington simply not care enough to act decisively and sanction such a bold new move? It seemed so to Mayor Maynard.

Maynard lost no time taking his complaints to the press. The headline for *The Washington Post* that day read: "Nome Mayor Attacks Capital for Inactivity."

"This bureaucracy stands idly by while our people suffer and die and while red-blooded men are willing to fly airplanes to our relief," Maynard said. "If Nome is compelled to wait until the Governor of Alaska considers that conditions here are really serious, Nome might as well abolish its Public Health Board, to govern our life and death from Juneau. . . ."

Bone's health official, Harry DeVighne, bristled at the attack: "Alarming reports sent out from Nome in criticism of official agencies are wholly unjustified," he told reporters.

". . . The territory is alertly watching the situation and while I believe that the delivery of the larger supply from Seattle would be safer by dog team than by any airplane available in the territory, the flight will be authorized if warranted by a crisis."

With that public statement, the governor's office sent a message to Wetzler directing him to round up more drivers for a second relay. Meanwhile, the train at Seward was ordered to idle at the station and wait for the serum, which was to arrive on board the *Admiral Watson* the next day, Saturday.

The U.S. Army, the U.S. Navy, and the airplane executives in Fairbanks, however, acting on an initiative begun by Maynard and perhaps fueled by news of Vera McDowell's death, continued to prepare for the flight. There was nothing the governor could do to stop them.

In Fairbanks, mechanics fitted skis to the plane and tuned the motor. Pilots Darling and Mackie stowed an extra propeller on board, along with "as many spare engine parts as weight will permit," sleeping bags, rifles, snowshoes, and camp equipment.

"If forced down," they told the North American Newspaper Alliance in an interview, "we will mush over the trail and connect with the dog teams [of the second relay]. . . . The antitoxin will not freeze unless we do. We will carry it in containers next to our bodies."

The two may have known a great deal about airplanes, but they knew very little about traveling even short distances in the Alaska wilderness without dogs.

In Seattle, at the behest of Washington officials, Commandant J.V. Chase of the Navy Yard at Bremerton ordered the minesweeper *Swallow* to prepare once again to head to the edge of the ice pack to aid the fliers in case they hit trouble on their way to Nome.

"It is most gallant of Darling," said another official, Dr. George Magruder, the head of the Public Health Service in Seattle, who coordinated the shipment of the 1.1 million units to Alaska. "The flight under the best of conditions is extremely hazardous. With an old plane . . . and in the dead of winter it is a perilous venture."

Although Chase's actions and Magruder's comments certainly encouraged those who argued on behalf of an air rescue, it was not clear how a sweeper would help if and when the rescue actually began. But that may not have been the point.

In addition, the army ordered the men of the Signal Corps to prepare fires along the route to guide the fliers, and in Nome, Captain Thomas Ross of the U.S. Lifesaving Crew began, with the help of his colleagues, to hack out a landing field on the Bering Sea in front of Nome. As far as Maynard, Sutherland, and Thompson were concerned, everything was in place for a flight—except Governor Bone's authorization.

On Saturday, February 7, with the serum due to arrive by ship late that evening, Bone reversed himself and sent a message to Wetzler authorizing him to divert half of the 1.1 million units when it arrived by train the next day. It was clear that he was taking the action under duress, most likely as a consequence of a report of yet another diphtheria case. The officials in Nome were in "hysteria," Bone said in his message to Wetzler. "There is no emergency that justifies such a hazard. However, I sincerely trust that nothing will go wrong."

Early Sunday afternoon, as the second batch of serum headed by train toward Nenana and then on to Fairbanks, Darling and Mackie went to the hangar where the *Anchorage* was stored to make last-minute preparations for the flight. They were both wearing several layers of fur clothing, and on their faces they had smeared petroleum grease a quarter of an inch thick to protect them from the cold. They wore close-fitting chamois helmets, with peepholes for their eyes and nostrils, and between them they had a single parachute—a problem, one newspaper reported, that would be "solved between themselves."

Finally, they packed two thermos bottles filled with hot liquid, a bar of chocolate, bullion cubes, beans, rice, flour, an ax, and extra fur robes.

It was time to start the engine. The serum was due by train some time soon.

Mackie and Darling heaved themselves into the open cockpit. A crowd had gathered to watch them. A volunteer mechanic by the name of Richard Lynch moved toward the front of the plane to spring the propeller.

It was about 40 below. Lynch, who had borrowed Mackie's new overcoat to help keep him warm, stepped up to the propeller, swinging the blade down hard. Unexpectedly, the propeller caught on the first try and the engine sprang to life. (It was a rare event for the propellers of the Fairbanks fleet to catch at the first try.)

Caught off guard by his success, Lynch, in trying to back away, slipped on the snow and got Mackie's overcoat caught in the first revolution of the blade. He was hurled 10 feet into the air. Luckily, Mackie's coat ripped and Lynch came crashing down to the ground, injuring his knee and breaking $10 worth of new tobacco pipes that had been in Mackie's coat pocket.

The engine roared to life and kept roaring. Mackie spent several minutes trying to idle it down but he could not. A mechanic standing at the back of the plane, holding down the tail while the engine ran at full speed, began to suffer from frostbite on his face. The slipstream created by the propeller was causing air to condense, forming a coat of ice on the fuselage and the tail, as well as on the mechanic's face.

In the cockpit, Darling's feet grew numb while Mackie, fiddling with the engine, lost feeling in his hands. The problem preventing them from regulating the engine was a broken radiator shutter, which caused the engine to overheat.

They would have to improvise another shutter, but that would take time, and the light in the sky was fading. The decision was made to call off the flight for the day. As the pilots and mechanics unloaded the provisions from the plane and began to work on a new shutter, a musher by the name of A. C. Olin left Nenana at 5:00 P.M. by dog team, headed for Tolovana. Packed in his sled were half of the 1.1 million units of antitoxin.

Despite the day's fiasco, Mackie and Darling were not dismayed. The two men told reporters that evening that they would be ready to take off the next day and land in Nome before Wednesday.

On Monday morning, the radiator again was troublesome. Not enough alcohol and glycerine had been added to the water in the radiator and it had frozen.

But Mackie remained confident.

"Our plane will pass the dogs before we have been in the air for two hours," he predicted. But on Tuesday the pilots again failed to get off the ground.

Finally, *News-Miner* editor Thompson, for whom the daring air rescue had meant so much, faced the truth. There would be no air rescue. And in that decision, Governor Bone was vindicated.

To HIS credit, Bone had not relied uncritically on the information being fed him from Fairbanks. From the first news of the epidemic, the governor had been receiving only glowing reports from Fairbanks on the plane's condition and the pilots' experience. Roy Darling had personally told Bone that the flight would be "no great difficulty," adding that "in the event of a forced landing we would expect nothing more serious than the delay incident to reaching nearest point of communication." But few forced landings were smooth in Alaska, especially at 50 or 60 degrees below, in blizzard conditions.

There was more than just a healthy skepticism influencing Bone's decisions. Despite the fears of Welch and others that the epidemic was not close to being under control, and that it might yet spread beyond the environs of Nome, Bone had quietly met with his health adviser, Harry DeVighne. After looking at all the information coming in from Nome, he concluded that the number of recoveries was beginning to outpace the number of new cases in Nome.[2] The situation was not dire enough to warrant the extreme risk of total failure involved in the flight.

Even more important, Bone had recently received a telegram from an aide in Anchorage who had done some research into Darling and the plane. The message made clear that the last time Darling had been in the air was after his crash, six years before. In addition, the *Anchorage*'s engine had six hundred hours of service life, more than half of which had already been used up. Partly because the motor had so many hours on it, the plane was capable of doing only 60 mph. This meant it would take several hours longer than Thompson had anticipated to reach Nome and would require more than one stop to refuel, increasing the risk of an accident on landing or takeoff.

This information had been crucial in Bone's decision to avoid using the *Anchorage* in any but the most desperate situation. It is unclear even today why he finally capitulated. Perhaps by that point he was already convinced that whether or not the plane made it, the epidemic was winding down and the half of the second shipment that would be going by dogsled might be enough to wipe it out altogether. Or perhaps he knew that the *Anchorage* would never get off the ground.

In defeat, Thompson was neither defiant nor dismissive of the great accomplishments of his opponents. To his credit, he struck just the right tone.

2. The precise number of deaths from the Nome epidemic remains a matter of conjecture. Some documents put the official death toll at six, others at five. Welch once said he thought it was probably seven, with a total of seventy confirmed cases overall. But in an interview with his hometown New Haven newspaper, he indicated the death toll could have been much higher.

"There must have been many more," Welch told a *New Haven Evening Register* reporter, October 9, 1925. "I imagine there were at least a hundred cases among the Natives and no telling how many deaths in the Eskimo camps outside of the city. The Natives have a habit of burying their children without reporting the death."

"We believe in the airship and we believe in the dog . . . ," he would write in a *News-Miner* editorial that evening.

> We know that even an ordinary airship can make 60 miles an hour and we know that a dog cannot. Where the dog has it over the airship is that the dog . . . knows nothing about horizons, visibilities, temperatures, gasoline—all he knows is to obey his master's voice and marche. . . . The burden of proof is today on the airship. The dogs are running and every hour getting closer to the goal. The airship will go when it can, but the dog seems to go whether he can or not. We take our hat off to THE DOG.

Indeed, by the time Thompson's editorial appeared, the second relay—which included many of the drivers from the first—had already safely left the town of Ruby, a little over a third of the way to Nome. The second run had also been difficult, with heavy snowstorms. The drivers were forced to break trail for much of the way.

Finally, on February 15, in the middle of a blizzard, Ed Rohn brought the second shipment of serum to Nome after a ninety-mile run. His lead dog, Star, was in the basket of his sled. Star had fallen through a fissure while crossing Golovin Bay and was badly injured.

Thompson could be magnanimous in defeat because the setback could only be temporary. The day of the dogs would soon pass into history. The race to save an arctic town did for Alaska what he could never have done with all his harangues—it focused the attention of the entire country on his territory.

ON FEBRUARY 2, the same day that Gunnar Kaasen drove his team into Nome, President Coolidge signed the Airmail Act of 1925, otherwise known as the Kelly Act. The legislation, which had been introduced three years earlier by Representative Clyde M. Kelly of Pennsylvania, had accelerated through Congress in the past few weeks. Private air companies would now be allowed to bid on contracts for mail delivery.

Airplane companies in Alaska were free to compete against the dog teams for mail contracts. Over the course of the next several years, technology on the ground and in the air improved and, increasingly, the small aviation companies that began to spring up in Alaska beat out the dogs in the bidding wars for the mail.

Within a decade of the serum run, there were several permanent air-mail runs. In 1938, Charlie Biederman marked the end of an era on the upper Yukon River when he delivered the last batch of contract mail by dog team. His sled would eventually be donated to the Smithsonian's Postal Museum. "Now the Dog and the Driver have arrived at the End of the Trail—the new way, the Airplane and the Pilot, takes over the task," said one Alaskan postmaster at the time. "The Dog has had its day. May the Airplane and the Pilot be as faithful."

By 1941, planes covered fifty-six routes while dog teams covered only ten, and by the early 1960s only a single dog route remained in Alaska: it was on St. Lawrence Island, about 150 miles off the coast in the Bering Sea. The postman was Chester Noongwook, who drove his team fifty miles to the landing strip where the air-mail plane touched down. His last run took place in January 1963.

COMMERCIAL AVIATION expanded in Alaska along with the air-mail routes. Operators took in extra income by flying passengers along with the regular mail. One of the first companies in the area to discover the potential windfall was Fairbanks Air. In June 1925, Noel Wien made the first round-trip commercial flight between Fairbanks and Nome. Wien flew an "aerial limousine," a five-passenger Fokker with an enclosed cabin that had upholstered seats and curtains.

On his first return flight, Wien carried the latest issue of the *Nome Nugget*, wrapped especially for the occasion and marked: "First Trip Air Mail Nome-Fairbanks. Courtesy Fairbanks Airplane Corp."

The trip had taken seven hours. It was a proud moment for "Wrong Font" Thompson, the feisty editor and aviation advocate. This would be one of the last causes he would ever fight for Alaska.

On January 4, 1926, Thompson died of pneumonia. He was in his early sixties.

As air-mail and passenger service gradually expanded across the state, the network of trails that had once been the territory's pride became overgrown, roadhouses were abandoned, and many of the smaller towns vanished. In 1931, when Charles Lindbergh and his wife flew over the Seward Peninsula and landed in a sheltered harbor south of Nome, Anne Morrow Lindbergh noticed the sad state of the roadhouses along the coast. "Dilapidated shingled buildings they were," she remembered. "Fast becoming useless; for the airplane . . . is replacing the dog team. It is cheaper per pound to fly."

The death knell for the heritage of dogsledding in Alaska came in the late 1950s, when the modern snowmobile was invented. The vehicles quickly became popular in Alaska and the dog teams became almost a novelty in many villages. By the 1960s, the sled dog population in most Alaskan villages was smaller than the number of "iron dogs," according to one sled dog historian.

The introduction of modern technology made it much easier to get in and out of Alaska, but without the territory's vast network of trails, travel inside it was dependent on airline schedules and specific routes. A snowmobile could only go so far on a tank of gas. Besides, it weighed several hundred pounds, was hard to maneuver over ravines or across creeks, and the engine became cranky at 20 degrees below zero. Over weak ice, a snowmobile could be a dangerous vehicle, and very hard to free up once icebound.

By 1970, travel over most of Alaska's trails was a thing of the past. A local historian, Dorothy Page, had joined forces with a sled dog enthusiast named Joe Redington and together they decided to create a race that would serve as a tribute to the dogs and their contribution to early Alaska.

For years, they had been aware that the trails were disappearing, and that an entire way of life was being eradicated. They conceived of a dog team race like no other, a homage to a disappearing world.

The first race to go all the way from Anchorage to Nome took place in 1973, and it has since been held every year on the first Saturday of March. It is called the Iditarod. The race covers what had once been a vital freight route between Anchorage and Nome, passing through the old Iditarod Mining District. (The route had fallen into disuse over time, particularly after the completion of the Seward to Fairbanks Railroad.)[3]

Iditarod is the name of a river on which the town was built when gold was discovered in 1907, and the word comes from an Athabaskan Indian term that has been translated as "a distant place" and "clear water." The exact definition has never been very clear. The race travels across the westernmost portion of the serum route: from Ruby to Nome in even years and from Kaltag to Nome in odd years.

In 1975, Alaska again showed its enthusiasm for dogsledding by holding a reenactment of the serum run. Many of the sons of the original drivers took part in the relay, which took six days longer than in 1925.

Today, the Iditarod is a $4 million industry that enjoys the support of a number of corporate sponsors and uses high-tech equipment along a trail that is broken out every year by volunteers on snowmobiles. Where once it had taken a front-runner three weeks to reach Nome, it now takes between eight and ten days. Today, a team of Siberians would not even place in the running. The sled dogs that run in the Iditarod are mostly Alaskan Huskies, which are even smaller and swifter than the Siberian. The Alaskan Husky is not a registered breed but a bloodline of racing dogs, a hybrid bred for speed. (That speed has come at the expense of some cold-weather adaptations, which is why many of the dogs need coats and booties, as well as a greater amount of food, when they race.) The winning dogs of the Iditarod are generally crossbreeds of Siberian Huskies and other Native dogs mixed in with speedier Irish Setters, English pointers, and German shorthairs. According to Raymond Coppinger, professor

3. The first incarnation of the Iditarod was in 1967, in celebration of America's purchase of Alaska. That year also marked the death of Leonhard Seppala. Acknowledging his contribution to Alaska, the twenty-five-mile contest was called the Iditarod Trail Seppala Memorial Race.

of biology at Hampshire College, "when the distance is over ten miles, modern racing sled dogs are the fastest animals in the world." With a person and sled attached, these dogs can run 3.2-minute miles for nearly twenty-five miles over a varied terrain that includes hills, curves, and woods.

"Siberians are kind of like racing an old sports car," says Bob Thomas, president of the International Siberian Husky Club. "You know the newer models are faster but there's just something special about driving that old classic."

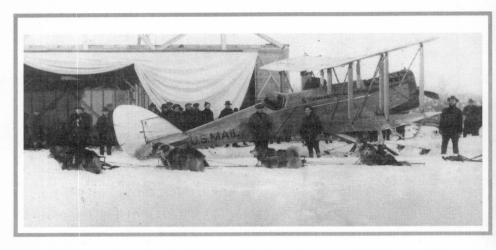

Every dog must have his day. A 1924 photograph of Carl Ben Eielson's plane
captioned: "Alaska's Mail Service: Yesterday and Today."
(Anchorage Museum of History and Art/B72.88.45)

EPILOGUE

End of the Trail

"No, there is no gold; there is no purse for the winner. They don't get a cent. . . . We give medals during the war for the taking of human life. So why not let Congress vote some congressional medals for these men who sacrificed to save the most precious of human life. A child!"
— WILL ROGERS, FEBRUARY 8, 1925

ON SATURDAY, February 21, two weeks after Kaasen reached Nome with the serum, the quarantine was lifted. The Dream Theatre celebrated by inviting everyone in town over twelve to a free double bill of the Harold Lloyd comedy *Grandma's Boy* and *Shirley of the Circus*, a Shirley Mason five-reeler. James Clark, who ran the moviehouse, decided to wait a few more weeks before letting the younger kids in.

Beyond Nome, the celebration began much earlier. Within hours of Kaasen's arrival, the local stringers for Associated Press, International News Service, Pathé News, and other news organizations had sent out dispatches over the radio and telegraph announcing the victory of man and dog over the worst that nature could throw at them. Despite the storm, they said, the serum had gotten through.[1] By the

---

1. Over the next few years, cases continued to crop up in Nome, but there was no longer any panic because the town had a fresh supply of serum on hand. Forty-three people contracted the disease in 1926 and there were about a dozen cases in 1928 and 1929.

following day, readers all over the country were reading about the men and dogs who had been "goaded on to the last measure of their strength" to reach Nome.

"Science made the antitoxin that is in Nome today," cheered *The New York Sun* in an editorial, "but science could not get it there. All the mechanical transportation marvels of modern times faltered in the presence of the elements. . . . Other engines might freeze and choke, but that oldest of all motors, the heart, whose fuel is blood and whose spark is courage, never stalls but once."

From the White House, President Coolidge sent out letters of commendation, while the Senate stopped its work to pay tribute to "that classic, heroic dog team relay that carried the life-saving antitoxin to the suffering, dying people of the little town of Nome, way

---

The 1925 epidemic had held the nation in thrall for nearly two months, and the publicity surrounding the race helped to galvanize the national campaign to inoculate children against the disease. In 1924, a researcher at the Pasteur Institute created an acceptable diphtheria vaccine that provided several years of active immunity—as opposed to the shorter duration of a passive immunity. The vaccine involved disarming the toxin with a chemical while enabling the body to stimulate the natural production of antibodies. Before this, scientists had tried to stimulate the natural immune system with "toxin-antitoxin," a balanced blend of poison and attenuated toxin. The public was wary of the new vaccine, but accepted it eventually. The serum run had been a reminder of how unpredictable and dangerous the disease could be, and it had helped raise awareness nationwide.

The United States was finally able dramatically to reduce the number of diphtheria cases; by 1945, there were only about 19,000 cases a year, and by 1960, fewer than 1,000.

Today, there are a handful of cases a year, and the victims are almost always people who have fallen through the cracks of the national health care system and have not been properly immunized. American children are forbidden to attend school or day care without immunization; since the 1940s, the vaccine has been incorporated into the DPT shot, which also offers protection against pertussis and tetanus.

Although diphtheria is now rare in the United States, it has made a comeback in other parts of the world, particularly where war and corruption have devastated the health infrastructure. In the past ten years, Russia and several former Soviet states have fought off outbreaks of the disease.

out there on the bleak coast of the Bering Sea," as Washington senator Clarence Cleveland Dill inserted in the record.

The pharmaceutical firm H. K. Mulford gave out twenty gold
medals, one for each driver on the first relay. The Alaskan government also gave each of them $25 as well as a citation stamped with the
territorial gold seal.

Public response was overwhelming. The *Seattle Times* ran a public
subscription fund to raise money for the drivers and the dogs, and the
proceeds were divided equally among them. Dozens of letters and
poems addressed to "Balto" began to pour into Nome's post office.
Local schoolchildren did their best to reply to most of them; the
Nome Nugget received more poems than it could print and issued an
apology. A churchman in Pasadena, California, sent in a poem enti-
tled "Balto, Hero of the Snows," and several writers in Atlanta sent in
their own rhyming tributes to the dog. Paeans were received as well
by state and federal officials, including a demand by one New Jersey
resident that Nome be renamed Balto "in honor of Gunnar Kaasen's
famous lead dog."

The media realized that there was even more money to be made
from the courage of others. The wire photo service Pacific & Atlantic
arranged for a driver to deliver the first photographs and newsreel
footage of the relay. They were, in fact, reenactments of Kaasen's
arrival in Nome.

A veteran musher named John Hegness raced across Alaska and
then south to the ice-free ports, where he caught a steamship and
headed for Seattle. Three hundred miles north of Seattle, a seaplane
and small boat were waiting for him. Hegness, who had sealed the
film in a can, threw it overboard for the crew of the small boat to
retrieve from the waters and transport to the seaplane. The pictures
were flown to Seattle and rushed by car to the offices of the *Seattle
Times*. Hegness remained on board the ship and arrived several hours
later in time to see the first pictures of the serum run splashed across
a full-page extra of the evening edition of the *Seattle Times*, five weeks
after leaving Nome.

Within days of the run, offers also began to pour in from the movies, as well as from showmen and publicists of every kind. Because Kaasen was the first driver to reach Nome, the newspapers rushed to describe his and Balto's experience on the trail. Kaasen and his team became instant celebrities, and by late February 1925, they had a movie deal and a tour lined up and were on their way to the states. With Balto and the other dogs, Kaasen and his wife, Anna, traveled south to Seward, where they boarded the steamship *Alameda* for Seattle. It was the first time in twenty-one years that the quiet musher had left Nome, and by the time the ship reached Seattle, a hero's welcome awaited him. The Associated Press got a photo of Gunnar, Anna, and Balto on deck, and a crowd encircled them. Kaasen then greeted his old friend from Nome, Ralph Lomen, who was in Seattle at the time, and told him: "I was praying you'd be here to protect me." Moments later, he was lost in the crowd. "We've been here only 10 minutes and I've lost my husband already," Anna Kaasen complained. "I could start back to Nome right now and not feel so badly about it."

Weeks later, Kaasen and the dogs began their brief movie career. Hollywood producer Sol Lesser, who would later make Rin Tin Tin and Tarzan pictures, shot the dog and driver for a thirty-minute film called *Balto's Race to Nome*. Lesser wasted no time hiring Kaasen and his team to promote the movie, and soon they were touring venues on the West Coast. In Los Angeles, Mary Pickford sat with Balto on the steps of City Hall as the mayor placed a wreath of flowers around the dog's neck.

While Kaasen and the dogs were touring the West Coast, the parks commissioner of New York City announced that a statue of Balto would be erected in Central Park. It was a rare honor, normally accorded only to such luminaries as Christopher Columbus, William Shakespeare, and Alexander Hamilton. Donations poured in to build the statue and the well-known sculptor Frederick Roth began to design it. Kaasen finished up his Hollywood commitments and, under the auspices of another promoter, went on a nine-month-long vaudeville circuit of the states. (A pay dispute between Kaasen and Lesser had led to the sale of the team to the new promoter.) The tour ended in New York, where on December 16, Kaasen, dressed in a squirrel-fur parka and timber wolf–fur pants, attended the unveiling of the statue. Balto stood quietly by his side, displaying no interest in the ceremonies until two northern sled dogs brought back from the Yukon Territory broke from the crowd and tried to join them. Kaasen managed to prevent the dogs from getting into a fight.

After the unveiling, Kaasen reluctantly left the dogs behind with the promoter who had bought the team and traveled back to Alaska through Canada. He arrived in Nenana by train and immediately returned to his job hauling supplies. Earl Modini, the proprietor of the Independent Meat Market store in Nome, had ordered seventy-five cases of yeast, and Kaasen borrowed a dog team and transported them to Nome.

It had been almost a year since Kaasen had left Nome, and when he returned in February 1926 he found his small town transformed. While he was away, a bitter feud had developed over the attention he had received from the press. Some Nome residents were angry and jealous of the movie offers and accused Kaasen of intentionally bypassing the last driver, Ed Rohn. They said he was trying to capture for himself the glory that would fall on whichever musher delivered the serum to Welch's door. Kaasen's supporters defended him, arguing that he had been blinded by the ferocity of the blizzard and had missed the roadhouse at Solomon. Therefore, they argued, he had never received the message to halt the relay.

The facts may never be known. Most of the relay drivers and residents or other witnesses to the history of the run died without giving a full account. Kaasen, who was a man of few words, rarely spoke of it. The *Fairbanks Daily News-Miner* maintained that Kaasen was reluctant to go on tour and that Mayor Maynard had persuaded him.

"He would rather make his hard mush over again, day after day, than appear on the stage where every eye in the house would be staring at him," wrote William Thompson.

Even on tour, Kaasen seldom spoke to the press. One polite newspaper account in the *Seattle Post-Intelligencer* described him as having "the shrinking modesty so generally accepted as becoming of a man of strong deeds. . . . On his rugged face is written an expression of pained patience which seems to say: 'Ho hum! This business of being a film star isn't all it's cracked up to be.' "

The feud between the two camps simmered for years and was revived after Kaasen retired from mining and moved to Everett, Washington, in 1952. Six years later, a reporter again raised the question that Kaasen might have bypassed Solomon roadhouse on purpose.

"Nonsense," Kaasen snapped. "I was blind."

The interview was over.

At first, Leonhard Seppala chose to stay out of the fray. In the immediate aftermath of the run, he focused on finding Togo and another teammate. The dogs had picked up the scent of reindeer on their return to Nome and had broken free of their harnesses. For days, Seppala worried that Togo had been mistaken for a wolf and shot by a reindeer herder, or that he had gotten his foot caught in a fox trap, a fairly common fate of sled dogs.

Eventually, the two dogs wandered back to the kennel at Little Creek and were reunited with their worried owner.

Seppala praised Kaasen for making the tough trek to Nome, but he was less generous when Togo's contribution failed to be as celebrated as Balto's. He was outraged that several newspapers had incorrectly attributed Togo's trail achievements to Balto, and devastated when he learned that New York was about to put up a bronze effigy of the wrong dog.

Seppala had once said that "in Alaska, our dogs mean considerably more to us than those 'outside' can appreciate, and a slight to them is as serious a matter to their drivers as if a human being's achievements were overlooked." The lack of recognition afforded Togo was a serious and heart-wrenching blow to him.

"It was almost more than I could bear when the 'newspaper' dog Balto received a statue for his 'glorious achievements,'" Seppala wrote in his memoirs.

For the next several years, Seppala would go out of his way to remind the public that he and Togo had traveled farther than any of the other teams, and that their section of the route had been by far the most dangerous. Seppala even claimed it was Fox, not Balto, who had led Kaasen's team.[2]

Seppala had designated Fox as the leader of the second string and had accused reporters of failing to give the dog his due. Fox was a common name in Alaska, he explained. It would never have stood out in a headline, whereas Balto's name was a grabber.

Seppala was always offended by the statue of the "wrong dog," but in his memoirs he chose to backtrack from the graver accusations about Kaasen and Balto:

> I hope I shall never be the man to take away credit from any dog or driver who participated in that run. We all did our best. But when the country was roused to enthusiasm over the serum run driver, I resented the statue to Balto, for if any dog deserved special mention it was Togo. . . . At the time I left [for the run] I never dreamed that anyone could consider these dogs [the second string] fit to drive even in a short relay. . . . As to the leader, it was up to the driver who happened to be selected to choose any dog he liked, and he chose Balto.

Regardless of any possible justification, it was not in Seppala's nature to show disrespect for an Alaskan sled dog.

By fall 1926, Seppala had made his own plans to take his Siberian dogs on tour with the ultimate goal of racing in the Northeast. In October, he left Nome with Togo and forty-two other dogs on one of the last steamships sailing before the winter set in. At last Togo would

---

2. After the run, reports slowly came out in the press that suggested Balto may not have been the sole leader of Kaasen's team. Popular dog biographer Albert Payson Terhune, who met Kaasen and Balto during their U.S. tour, told the McKnaught Syndicate that according to these reports the initial leader of Kaasen's team had been felled by the brutal cold. Another lead dog was chosen, but he too was beaten by the storm. "Then Balto was put in the lead. He did not wear out and he did not quit. Not only did he keep the rest of his team up to their work, but he found and kept the trail." It is possible that Kaasen had to switch dogs around on the team. Mushers will attest that even good lead dogs often refuse to run into a gale.

receive the national recognition he deserved. Seppala and his Siberians made an astonishing number of promotional appearances. The tour took him from Seattle to California and across the midwestern states to the Northeast, a logistical feat that required the patience of a saint as well as enormous skill. It would have been hard to imagine anyone else in charge. He posed for photographs with Togo and the whole team in department stores and he appeared in a national ad campaign for Lucky Strike cigarettes. To the delight of his child fans and their parents, he would demonstrate what it was like to live in the Arctic and he lectured on Siberian dogs.

In town after town, Seppala paraded the whole team down Main Street. According to one report, he visited fifty midwestern towns in a whirlwind three-day jaunt. There was something larger than life about the diminutive Seppala. Wherever he went, he drew crowds so huge that the police often had to be brought in to maintain control. In Kansas City, some of the dogs were hurt when the crowd became too big, and during an event at a Detroit auditorium, spectators surged forward to see him in his fur parka and sealskin pants and almost trampled him. In one town, Seppala and his Siberians drew a larger crowd than President Coolidge had. Oddly, this man who had spent so much of his life in the company of dogs turned out to be a natural-born public speaker, combining playfulness with wry humor. He told one audience that his secret for staying in shape at the late age of fifty was that he neither smoked nor drank. Then, as he was turning somersaults and handsprings, two cigars fell out of his pocket. The crowd roared.

"They probably considered it all part of the show," a friend had said.

New York City was the last stop on the tour. With Togo at the lead, Seppala drove the serum run team to the top of the steps of City Hall, then up Fifth Avenue, and finally on a circuit through Central Park. There was a series of appearances at Madison Square Garden, where former Nome resident and current Garden manager Tex Rickard had arranged a ten-day exhibition. Before thousands of spectators, Seppala drove the team around the ice hockey rink, and the dogs were so excited they sped around the turns at top speed, crashing into the walls. During halftime at one game, the explorer Roald Amundsen went out on the ice to give a speech honoring Togo, and presented the animal with a gold medal. There was thunderous applause from the twenty thousand spectators. It was a fitting end to the tour, and when it was over Seppala was free to return to his great love, racing.

At the invitation of Arthur Walden of the Chinook Kennels in Wonalancet, New Hampshire, Seppala headed up to New England in January 1927 to participate in the burgeoning race circuit. Walden had been a dog freighter during the Klondike and Alaskan gold rushes and had returned to New Hampshire to become an enthusiastic promoter of sled dogs. He was instrumental in organizing the first race in New England in 1921 and the New England Sled Dog Club in 1924, and he was curious to know how his own line of dogs, the chinook, would stand up to Seppala's little Siberians. Walden's chinooks were renowned in the Northeast. They were flop-eared, tawny dogs with a mixed ancestry that included Canadian sled dog, St. Bernard, Belgian sheepdog, and German shepherd.

They appeared unbeatable until Seppala arrived.

Seppala and his Siberians blew the competition away. In his first race in Poland Springs, Maine, in January, Seppala beat out his host and the other competitors by more than seven minutes. The crowds were amazed at the appearance of this new team and the performance of the small dogs. The win was even more remarkable for the fact that his dogs were hardly conditioned from their tour of the United States, and Seppala had stopped mid-race to help untangle a competitor's dog team. The competitor was a Poland Spring socialite named Elizabeth Ricker, whose family owned the Poland Spring Resort and were sponsoring the race. Ricker was so impressed with Seppala's dogs that she not only replaced her dog team with a team of Seppala's Siberians but bought most of the remaining Siberians Seppala had brought with him from Alaska. Then, with Seppala as co-manager, Ricker opened up a kennel at the resort, and the two began to breed and sell the Siberians.

Seppala's participation in subsequent races led to a surge in the popularity of the sport in New England as well as to an increased interest in Siberian Huskies. In 1930, the American Kennel Club officially recognized the Siberian Husky as a breed.

(A large majority of registered huskies in the United States can boast of having Togo or one of his serum run teammates in their pedigree. Seppala had bolstered the original stock with more imports from Siberia. The last three ever to be imported from Siberia to the kennel came in 1930.)

For the next few years, after opening the kennel with Ricker, Seppala divided his time between Alaska and Maine. In March 1927, he made his first trip back to Alaska after his tour of the states. Togo had aged considerably since the serum run, and his vigor was now less pronounced. Seppala thought the trip back would be too much for the dog, so he decided to leave him behind with Ricker.

The serum run had been Togo's last long-distance race, one in which "he had worked his hardest and his best," and the dog was put into retirement to live out his final years. He spent most of his time by the fire in the living room of Ricker's home. "It was a sad parting on a cold gray March morning when Togo raised a small paw to my knee as if questioning why he was not going along with me," Seppala remembered.

It was probably for the best: Togo needed the rest. He was partially blind and the pain in his joints was worsening. On December 5, 1929, Seppala finally found the courage to put Togo to sleep. He was sixteen years old.

"Every once in a while a dog breaks through the daily routine of feeding and barking and tugging at a leash, and for some deed of super-canine heroism wins the adoring regard of every one who hears of him," *The New York Times Magazine* wrote in a eulogy. ". . . His was the kind of life that catches men by the throat and sets them to hero worshipping."

Years after Togo's death, Seppala kept the dog's spirit alive. One reporter, writing about Seppala many years later, said that "in the depths of his keen gray eyes—lives a dog who will never leave."

"While my trail has been rough at times," Seppala wrote in his journal when he was eighty-one, "the end of the course seems pretty smooth, with downhill going and a warm roadhouse in sight. And when I come to the end of the trail, I feel that along with my many friends, Togo will be waiting and I know that everything will be all right."

Togo's body was placed on exhibit at the Yale Peabody Museum in New Haven, Connecticut, where it remained for decades. Finally, it was returned to Alaska. It can still be seen in a glass case at the Iditarod Trail Sled Dog Race Museum outside Anchorage.

WHILE TOGO lived out his well-deserved retirement in Maine, Balto and his teammates were on the other side of the country struggling to survive in Southern California. After their circuit of vaudeville acts in the states, the dogs had ended up in a sideshow in Los Angeles. For ten cents a ticket, a customer could walk into a stuffy backroom and see the animals. They sat there for several months, neglected and abused. Had it not been for George Kimble, a businessman from Cleveland who recognized them, Balto and the others would likely have succumbed to the atrocious conditions. Kimble struck a deal with the owner and agreed to buy the entire team for $2,000. He had two weeks to come up with the money.

He returned to Cleveland and began a campaign through the *Cleveland Plain Dealer* to rescue the dogs. The response was overwhelming. Children donated milk money at school and waitresses and factory hands passed around the collection plate at work. Shops, hotels, and a local kennel club chipped in generously, and by the tenth day of the drive Kimble had his cash.

On March 19, 1927, Balto and six other teammates—Fox, Sye, Billy, Tillie, Moctoc, and Alaska Slim—were given a hero's welcome as they paraded through downtown Cleveland. (The six other serum run teammates had already died or been sold.) In harness again, they pulled a sled rigged with wheels and driven by a former gold stampeder named Marye Berne. Thousands lined the streets, a band played, and the dogs marched to their new home at the Brookside Zoo (now the Metroparks Zoo). On their first day there, nearly fifteen thousand people came to see them.

Balto and the serum run team would live out their remaining days at the zoo. Fox, Moctoc, Tillie, Alaska Slim, and Billy were the first to die. Then, at the beginning of March 1933, the zookeeper announced that Balto was ailing and had little time left. He had become blind and was partially deaf, and the zookeeper turned the dog over to a local veterinarian and trustee of the Balto Committee, which had helped to oversee the care of Balto. A few days later, on March 14, Balto died.

Although the newspapers reported that he was eleven, he may in fact have been as old as fourteen. (Seppala had once claimed that Balto was six at the time of the run.) His body was preserved and displayed at Cleveland's Natural History Museum, where to this day it forms a part of the collection.

Now Sye was the only remaining member of Kaasen's serum run team. The old dog took his teammates' departure hard and there were reports that he howled out of loneliness. A year later, on March 25, 1934, Sye passed away. He was seventeen.

For the most part, the other drivers in the serum run returned to their everyday lives once the intense publicity faded. Wild Bill Shannon, who had been on a brief tour with Blackie, continued to drive the mail, hunt, and run his traplines. He once said during a visit to the states: "This hero business is big blah . . . I want to get back [home] where they shake hands and know how to fry bacon."

A few years later, he was attacked and killed by a bear. Anna Shannon moved to Healy, a small village on the railroad, and there she set up a general store and continued to live the life of a pioneer.

"I wouldn't take a million dollars for the things I have done, and that I have learned," she once said.

Relatively little is known about the Native drivers who covered nearly two thirds of the run. Few reporters or moviemakers wanted to hear their story. For the most part, Alaska's Natives were considered a part of the landscape, regardless of the fact that they spoke the same language, held down jobs, and contributed to the economy. They were capable of the same acts of great and simple heroism as the white man, and they were not boastful about it. By and large, they were quiet and humble people who would go out of their way to help another human being in distress. Their Native tradition put a premium on cooperation.

For many of the Natives, a simple thank-you was sufficient. "I got more in gratitude from one lady at Nome City than I ever would have got in money from that race," said Charlie Evans, who ran through the ice fog and lost two dogs in the sprint from Bishop Mountain to Nulato.

"During the serum run I was just over 20," said Edgar Kallands, whose hands were frozen to the sled on his run from Tolovana to Manley Hot Springs. "Time stands still at that time, the prime of life. It was just an every day occurrence as far as we were concerned."

In the 1970s, during a surge in interest to preserve Alaska's history, stories about the Native drivers' heroism began to emerge. By then, many of them had died and the memories of those still alive had faded. Nevertheless, their role in the run was acknowledged, and they began to gain the recognition that had eluded them for so many years.

In the early years of the now-famous annual Iditarod race, reporters sought out the original drivers, and race officials bestowed on them the honorary "Number 1" position.

In 1985, on the sixtieth anniversary of the serum run, President Ronald Reagan sent each of the three surviving drivers a letter of recognition: honors went to Charlie Evans, Edgar Nollner, and Bill McCarty, an Athabaskan-Irish driver who traveled the route between Ruby and Whiskey Creek.

> Together with 19 others, you traveled across some of the world's cruelest miles to accomplish the impossible—and you did it in the name of humanity.[3]

3. The wording seems to have changed. This was the way it was reported in the Alaskan press. The actual text of Reagan's letter reads: ". . . after crossing some of the world's most forbidding miles. . . ."

They had, indeed, been the cruelest miles.

At the time of the run, the Interior was experiencing the coldest weather in twenty years. For many of the drivers—most of whom were barely twenty years old at the time and some as young as eighteen—the weather was far worse than anything they had experienced.

Edgar Nollner, who shared the run from Whiskey Creek to Bishop Mountain with his younger brother George, said he would not have gone out "if the situation had not been so dire. There is nothing to go out for when it's that cold."

In 1953, Edgar Nollner was once again called on to help, and he performed just as heroically. He had been gathering wood out in the wilderness with his dog team when he heard the crash of a U.S. Air Force plane. He discovered two injured crewmen next to the wreckage. It was 50 degrees below zero and they were both at risk of dying from hypothermia. Nollner built a fire for them, went back to get his friend Charlie Evans to help, and the two carried the wounded airmen to safety.

Nollner was the last survivor of the drivers on the first serum run. On January 18, 1999, he died of a heart attack at age ninety-four. He was survived by twenty-three children and more than two hundred grandchildren. In 1995, he told the Associated Press that he was surprised at all the attention and had never expected to become famous.

"I just wanted to help, that's all," he said.

Appendix A

Charlie Evans was Edgar Nollner's neighbor and brother-in-law, as well as an active member of the community. When the government neglected to send a teacher into town, Evans took the job. Asked what it was that he had taught, he replied, "right and wrong." In 1986, Evans donated his medal and certificate to the University of Alaska Museum. He died the following year, on July 22, at age eighty-four. He and his wife had thirteen children, six of whom died in early childhood.

Myles Gonangnan remained in Unalakleet all his life. He drove the mail from Unalakleet to Kotzebue for several years and helped interpret for the pastor at the local church. He died in April 1967 at the age of eighty-one.

Henry Ivanoff, who passed the serum to Seppala outside Shaktoolik after his dogs got into a fight, would die a few years after the serum run. He drowned at sea in 1934 after a storm wrecked the mailboat he was piloting north of Nome. His grandson, Henry "Gus" Johnson, ran the Iditarod in 1980, finishing twentieth in a field of sixty-one.

Gunnar and Anna Kaasen never had children but lived their remaining years in Everett, Washington, close to their great-nieces and -nephews. Gunnar led a quiet life, highlighted by long walks and trips with the children to buy vanilla ice cream at the store. He rarely spoke to them about the serum run, despite a constant peppering of questions. "I'm going to tell you this once and once only," he told one great-niece, Janice Weiland. "If it wasn't for Balto, I wouldn't be alive today."

Although he rarely referred to the run, his relatives were sure that Kaasen was proud of his role and that of Balto. Throughout his life, he kept on the living-room wall an old movie poster from his Hollywood days that showed him standing in his trail clothes next to Balto. Kaasen died of cancer in Everett in 1960, at the age of seventy-eight.

Edgar Kallands also stayed in Alaska. He carried mail, ran traplines, traded his beaver skins for fish for his dogs, and worked during the summer on the steamboats. Knee surgery in 1958 put an end to his work with the dogs. As a child, Kallands's best friend had been a puppy, and his dogs had often been his closest companions. When his knee went bad, he had to say good-bye to one of his greatest passions: "You had to be able to walk with dogs. Because if there's lots of new snow, you have to put on snowshoes and walk ahead of the dogs for long hours. When you get on snowshoes it means lots of work."

His last lead dog was Rover, a dog so attached to Kallands that he refused to pull for anyone else. Kallands died in December 1981 at the age of seventy-seven. He had four children and several grandchildren.

Bill McCarty trapped and fished most of his life in Ruby and raised ten children with his wife. Years after the serum run, he met a woman who had been in Nome during the epidemic and who recognized McCarty as one of the drivers. She thanked him for saving her life. "It made me feel good to know I had done some people good," McCarty said. In the 1950s, McCarty went blind from exposure to DDT and his lifestyle changed. Up until his death in 1989 at age eighty-five, the outdoorsman longed to return to the woods and to his subsistence lifestyle. According to his nephew, Bill always considered his role in the serum run as "a kind of normal operation."

George Nollner, who had sung an Athabaskan love song as he pulled into Bishop Mountain, was not so lucky as his brother Edgar. In 1930, he broke through the ice near Galena while traveling across the Yukon River with his team of four dogs. The sled went under first, and then he disappeared.

"They pulled them three dead dogs out and the sled, but my brother was gone," Edgar Nollner said. "They brought that one dog back but he hollered and hollered so bad because my brother went under they had to shoot him. Every night he hollered. It was my brother's lead dog."

Leonhard Seppala retired from Alaska and moved to Seattle in 1947, but he remained tireless and agile. At the age of eighty, he drove a dogsled into the city for a March of Dimes publicity campaign, "smiling, hearty and proud as ever." The organization had planned to kick off the event with a hydroplane but a snowstorm got in the way.

Seppala continued to extol the virtues of the Siberian Husky (their intelligence, speed, and stamina), and he was considered by many to be the patron saint of dogsledding. He donated his sled, his old goldmining equipment, and his fur clothes to a museum near his hometown in Norway. He died on January 28, 1967, at the age of eighty-nine. In his lifetime, Seppala logged an estimated 250,000 miles by dogsled.

IN THE years following the serum run, many of Nome's sourdough residents moved on. In 1928, Hammon superintendent Mark Summers and his family transferred to Fairbanks. Seppala and his family also moved to the Interior capital that same year for the company. Mayor George Maynard died in August 1939. He had been editor and manager of the *Nome Nugget* until the very end.

Emily Morgan remained at her post, rising to the level of hospital superintendent. It is not known when she left Nome. Her role in the serum run had been praised in the press and in the early 1970s one reporter described her as the "Angel of the Yukon." Morgan died on May 9, 1960, at the age of eighty-two.

Curtis Welch and his wife, ***Lula***, left Nome several months after the run, in September 1925. They had intended to stay Outside on vacation for a full year, but in early May the government called Welch back to take charge of a riverboat that was heading down the Yukon for a medical survey of the Natives living along the route. By September 1927, the Welches were back in Nome, where they stayed for two more years until Welch's health deteriorated to the extent that they had to move to a warmer climate. They settled in Santa Barbara, California.

"Northwestern Alaska is a young man's country," Welch wrote in his journal; ". . . a physician's calls must be made on foot . . . a walk of a mile or two at night, in a blizzard, with the temperature 20 or 30 below zero. . . . It is no job for an old man."

Over the next few years, the Welches would return in the summer to fill in for the town doctor while he was on vacation or to see friends. In the states and in Alaska, the reluctant Welch continued to be hailed as a hero, as essential a figure as the drivers had been. "In spite of his protestations, Curt really did like the attention," Lula said.

A close examination of Nome's medical crisis suggests that Welch erred by not identifying the disease early enough, and some blamed him for at least some of the deaths. Death records show that diphtheria was present in Nome as early as September 1924 with the death of a four-year-old boy named William Rothacker. Welch had written on the boy's death certificate that the cause of death was tonsillitis, which he later changed to diphtheria. If William Rothacker had indeed been diphtheria's first victim, this would predate Welch's official report and suggest that the disease had been present in Nome longer than the doctor had admitted to authorities. Had Welch tested the outdated serum on one of the earlier suspected cases, he would have known definitively that the serum was stable and effective, and he might have saved more lives. It should be noted, however, that diphtheria was hard to diagnose, more so without proper medical equipment, and Welch was certainly ill equipped. Just two months after the serum run, the U.S. Surgeon General offered to send him laboratory equipment so that he could diagnose outbreaks of diphtheria and other diseases.

The health official congratulated Welch on his handling of the epidemic and praised "the very commendable way in which you let the newspaper men do the talking and held the even tenor of your way. It has been a source of much gratification to the Public Health Service to have had such an able representative as yourself at one of our farthermost outposts."

Dr. Welch's last trip to Nome appears to have been in the summer of 1933, when he filled in once more for the town physician.

Lula's memoirs drop some hints about her husband's mood swings that suggest possible manic depression or alcoholism. After a long period of ill health, Dr. Welch died on December 14, 1948, at the age of seventy. The cause of death, according to his death certificate, was a morphine overdose, self-administered.

BY 1925, NOME had already lost much of the splendor of its gold rush years, and nature would make matters worse. A series of floods and storms knocked down many of the buildings on Front Street, and a 1934 fire destroyed much of the town. The Maynard Columbus Hospital survived the conflagration but burned to the ground during a blizzard in 1948, although the nurses' quarters remain intact to this day.

"Nome is on a slow retreat," said one resident, Edward Sheriff Curtis, in 1927. "We know each year will be a little worse than the one before."

Curtis's words captured the sentiment of the time. For a while, some residents considered relocating the town up Anvil Creek to safer ground, or seventy-three miles northwest to Teller, an abandoned reindeer station with a natural harbor. But despite what it has been forced to endure, Nome has survived. After every natural disaster, its residents chose to stay and rebuild. One resident has called it the town "that would not die."

In 1974, a storm nearly demolished Nome once again. It inflicted more than $30 million in property damage and was considered the worst in the town's history. A fortified sea wall, engineered by the U.S. Army, now helps to control the storm surge waves, but nothing can temper the blizzards or hold back the ice. Each year, winter descends on Nome in much the same fashion as it did in 1925.

Today, some 3,500 people live in Nome and the options for reaching the town are almost as few as they were in the 1920s. There are no roads or railroad lines. There are some passenger ships in summer; in winter, flights are frequent but are often grounded by bad weather. Most of those who arrive by dogsled are Iditarod racers.

With the start of the new millennium, however, Nome has once again acquired a certain cachet, albeit of a special kind. Some twenty thousand people visit the town every summer to see the vestiges of one of America's last gold stampedes.

Nome is a good show: there are still old dredges and buckets rusting on the beach alongside railroad ties pushed up out of the tundra. Dreamers still come to Nome to try their luck, camping out on the beach in tents. They bring modern contraptions to mine for gold, and they'll occasionally head up the creek with a pan and shovel.

Others simply come to take in the view and to experience life at the edge of the Bering Sea.

Appendix B

THE 1925 SERUM RUN PARTICIPANTS

The following is the generally accepted order of the mushers in the first serum run, as well as the mileage they covered.

	Musher	Relay Leg	Distance
Jan. 27–28	Bill Shannon	Nenana to Tolovana	52 miles
Jan. 28	Edgar Kallands	Tolovana to Manley Hot Springs	31 miles
Jan. 28	Dan Green	Manley Hot Springs to Fish Lake	28 miles
Jan. 28	Johnny Folger	Fish Lake to Tanana	26 miles
Jan. 29	Sam Joseph	Tanana to Kallands	34 miles
Jan. 29	Titus Nikolai	Kallands to Nine Mile Cabin	24 miles
Jan. 29	Dave Corning	Nine Mile Cabin to Kokrines	30 miles
Jan. 29	Harry Pitka	Kokrines to Ruby	30 miles
Jan. 29	Bill McCarty	Ruby to Whiskey Creek	28 miles
Jan. 29	Edgar Nollner	Whiskey Creek to Galena	24 miles
Jan. 30	George Nollner	Galena to Bishop Mountain	18 miles
Jan. 30	Charlie Evans	Bishop Mountain to Nulato	30 miles
Jan. 30	Tommy Patsy	Nulato to Kaltag	36 miles
Jan. 30	Jackscrew	Kaltag to Old Woman Shelter	40 miles
Jan. 30–31	Victor Anagick	Old Woman Shelter to Unalakleet	34 miles
Jan. 31	Myles Gonangnan	Unalakleet to Shaktoolik	40 miles
Jan. 31	Henry Ivanoff	Shaktoolik to Seppala handoff	
	Leonhard Seppala[1]	Shaktoolik to Golovin	91 miles
Feb. 1	Charlie Olson	Golovin to Bluff	25 miles
Feb. 1	Gunnar Kaasen	Bluff to Nome	53 miles

Total Miles: 674 miles

Total Time: 127 hours 30 minutes (5½ days

1. Leonhard Seppala drove 170 miles from Nome to Shaktoolik to meet the serum for a total of 261 miles in the first serum run, the longest distance in the whole run. On one day he covered 84 miles.

Acknowledgements

This book would not have been possible without the resources, support, and hospitality of many people and institutions across the United States during the three years we spent researching and writing. At the University of Alaska, Fairbanks, we are particularly grateful to Professor Terrence Cole of the history department. We also thank Syun-Ichi Akasofu, director of the International Arctic Research Center; Julia Triplehorn, librarian of the Keith B. Mather Library at the Geophysical Institute; and library assistant Ann Wood. We are also indebted to the dedicated staff at the university's Elmer E. Rasmuson Library: Robyn Russell, Dr. William Schneider, Dr. Susan Grigg, Caroline Atuk, Peggy Asbury, Richard Veazey, Rose Speranza, and Dirk Tordoff.

Ted Fathauer, lead forecaster of the National Weather Service in Fairbanks; four-time Iditarod champion Susan Butcher; sea-ice expert Dr. William Stringer; and Dermot Cole, reporter for the *Fairbanks Daily News-Miner*, were all generous with their time and help. To the ever-patient Campbell family in Tanana, thank you for the firsthand experience driving dogs in bush Alaska; and thanks to Dan O'Neill and Sarah Campbell for recounting their trip by dog team over the entire serum run trail.

We found a warm welcome wherever we traveled in Alaska. We would especially like to thank Richard K. Nelson for his inspiration; Diane Brenner and Kathleen Hertel of the Anchorage Museum of History and Art; Igor Kripnick of the Arctic Studies Center; Penny Rennick of the Alaska Geographic Society; Judy Skagerberg at the Alaska State Archives; Bea Shephard of the Methodist Church

Archives; Anne Laura Wood of the Alaska State Library; Mike Zaidlic and Donna Redding at the Bureau of Land Management; Dr. Robert Fortuine of the University of Alaska, Anchorage; Bruce Merrell of the Loussac Library; Joanne Potts of the Iditarod Trail Committee, Inc.; and Benoni Nelson at the Knik Museum and Mushers Hall of Fame.

Descendants of both Leonhard Seppala and Gunnar Kaasen offered freely of their time and memories. We would like to thank the many relatives of Gunnar Kaasen in both America and Norway, especially Jack Strege, Janice Weiland, and Stein Kaasen. We also thank the late Sigrid Seppala-Hanks and Bill Hanks for their assistance.

Nome of 1925 could not have been brought to life without help from many longtime residents such as Ruthmarie McDowell, Vesta Polsen, and Jean Summers-Wolf. As all researchers into Nome find out sooner or later, the many members of the Walsh clan were both gracious and informative. Our guide and host in Nome, fourth-generation Nome resident Cussy Kauer, was indispensable. She helped us in so many ways, often from 5,000 miles away, that we could never adequately thank her. Her Nome Cemetery Project, which city councilman Stan Andersen pushed through, was particularly vital to our efforts to reconstruct the epidemic. Others in Nome who helped were Deborah L. Redburn, John Handeland, Laura Samuelson, Lana Harris, Leslie Simone, Branson Tungiyan, Jerry A. Steiger, and Wes Perkins.

Researching the story of the serum run we also accumulated debts in England, Canada, and across the Lower 48. Many experts enthusiastically shared their knowledge with us, including the entire staff of the Cleveland Museum of Natural History, particularly their Balto expert, curator Steve Misencik; Sarah Bartash at the Cleveland Metroparks Zoo; Kenneth A. Ungermann, who wrote the classic account of the serum run more than forty years ago; Ed Blechner, whose devotion and tireless efforts to honor Togo's memory, upon finding his mount atop a refrigerator in a closet in Vermont, resulted in the dog hero's return to Alaska; Bob and Pam Thomas of the International Siberian Husky Club; Susan Carroll of the Merck Archives; Blaine Maley and Sara Cedar Miller at the Central Park Conservancy; Jonathan Kuhn at the New York City Parks Department; Barbara Narendra at Yale University's Peabody Museum; Polly C. Darnell and Barbara Rathburn of the Shelburne Museum in Vermont; John Parascandola and Marjorie Ciarlanti of the National Archives in Washington, D.C.; Elsie Chadwick of the Siberian Husky Club in Toronto; Julie Muhlstein of the *Everett Herald*; Jim Bowman of the Glenbow Archives in Calgary; Red Cross historian Jean Waldman; Herb Farmer at the USC Moving Image Archives; Gregory Malak of the Will Rogers Memorial Museum; and Ken Atherton, formerly of the UK Hydrographic Office. Others who were helpful include Julian "Bud" Lesser and Marjorie Fasman, the children of Sol Lesser; Jona Van Zyle; Dale and Nancy Wolff; Terris C. Howard; Matt Morgan; Lance McLean; and Wendy Fitzgerald.

The writing of a book is always a group effort, and we thank our many friends and family members who read draft after draft of the manuscript. In particular we thank our parents for their continued support, insight, home-cooked meals, and a refuge in the country for writing; we thank Ricky Fortunato, Dermot Cole, Terrence Cole, Dan O'Neill, and Bob and Pam Thomas for their careful reading, and Aly Sujo for his fine-tuning. Our cousin Ned Salisbury provided brilliant art direction; Adrienne Salisbury helped with photo and film research; and Harry Zernike was a merciless photo editor. The wonderful staff at Norton were behind the book from the beginning, particularly our editor, Starling Lawrence, and assistant editor, Morgen Van Vorst, as well as Louise Brockett, Jeannie Luciano, Felice Mello, Elizabeth Riley, and Bill Rusin.

Above all we want to thank the woman who has been there from the start, whose enthusiasm and editorial insight never wavered no matter what the condition of the trail, and who guided us along every step of the way, our friend and agent Susan Rabiner.

Finally we honor the "indomitable spirit" of the dog drivers and sled dogs of Alaska who together "carved a legend in the snow," and to the memory of all the dear dogs we've loved so well: Muffin, Major, Maoser, Magic, Piggy, Trixie, Jack, Lochy, Piper, Piper II, Cosmo, Frisbee, and Sasha.

Source Notes

To reconstruct the events of January 1925, we relied heavily on government documents, interviews, oral histories, and diaries. Wherever there were gaps in the record, we turned to secondary sources for guidance. Particularly helpful were Kenneth A. Ungermann's *The Race to Nome*, which contained interviews with many of the drivers; Leonhard Seppala's biography, *Seppala: Alaskan Dog Driver*, by Elizabeth M. Ricker; and a series of articles Seppala wrote with Raymond Thompson in *Alaska Sportsman*. A number of excellent trail descriptions by the late Don Bowers were also of great help. Memories are often fallible, and we sometimes found that our subjects remembered differing versions of the same event. Where accounts differed, we used our best judgment and tried to make informed decisions about what happened that fateful winter.

Prologue: Icebound

4 **Welch's life in Alaska:** Lula Welch as told to Marion Rankin Kennedy, "Northland Doctor's Wife," parts 1–11, *Alaska Sportsman* (May 1965–May 1966), provides extensive detail about Curtis and Lula Welch's life in Alaska; "Nome Doctor Hero New Haven Boy," *Hartford Courant*, February 7, 1925, includes letters Welch sent to his sister as well as interviews with his sister that open a window onto Welch's personality and feelings toward Alaska. See also Curtis Welch, "An Unfinished Memoir of Pioneer Days," 1939, June Metcalfe Collection, Rasmuson Library (hereafter cited as Rasmuson), University of Alaska, Fairbanks.

4 **an area as big as England, France, Italy:** Jim DuFresne, *Alaska: A Lonely Planet Travel Survival Kit* (Victoria, Australia: Lonely Planet Publications, 1997), 11.

4 **one would have to spend a lifetime:** Merle Colby, *A Guide to Alaska, Last American Frontier* (New York: Macmillan, 1945), vii.

5 **Front Street was never busier:** Frank Dufresne, *My Way Was North: An Alaskan Autobiography* (New York: Holt, Rinehart & Winston, 1966), portrays the frantic pace in Nome in the last days of fall, while letters from former Nome residents provide colorful detail of a town hunkering down for winter. Letters we received from Jean Summers-Wolf throughout 2001 were particularly helpful, as were interviews with the Walsh family.

7 **"an ocean of slush":** Dufresne, *My Way,* 27

7 **"It seemed to me that half":** Ibid.

7 **"tips of small torches":** Sally Carrighar, *Moonlight at Midday* (New York: Knopf, 1958), 70. Carrighar wrote in vivid detail about the natural beauty of Northwest Alaska.

8 **called it *ivu*:** Barry Lopez, *Arctic Dreams* (New York: Bantam Books, 1987), 176.

8 **a "great listening":** Carrighar, *Moonlight,* 71.

8 **"the breath out you":** Barrett Willoughby, "The Challenge of the Sweepstakes Trail," *American Magazine* (1926), James Wickersham Collection, Rasmuson.

8 **"as if an unseen hand":** John Wallace, "The People of Nome Were Scandalized," *Alaska Sportsman* (December 1939).

9 **not seen a single confirmed case:** Curtis Welch to U.S. Surgeon General Hugh Cumming, February 16, 1925, Report, National Archives, Record Group (RG) 90, U.S. Public Health Service, General Correspondence (hereafter cited as Welch Report). The report is Welch's official account of his actions during the epidemic.

9 **"Many cases have come under":** Welch Report.

Chapter One: Gold, Men, and Dogs

The chapter title comes from Alexander Allan's *Gold, Men and Dogs* (New York & London: G. P. Putnam's Sons, 1931). Allan wrote extensively about his life as a dog driver in the far north, including the training, feeding, breeding, and racing of his sled dogs.

12 **"a placer from a potato patch":** Quoted in Terrence Cole's history of Nome, *Nome: City of the Golden Beaches* (Anchorage: Alaska Geographic Society, 1984), 23.

13 **"You never saw a more":** Local historian Carrie McLain, recalled in her history, *Gold Rush Nome* (Portland, OR: Graphic Arts Center, 1969).

15 **"These men are mad"**: Loyal Lincoln Wirt, *Alaskan Adventures* (New York & London: Fleming H. Revell Co., 1937), 13. Considering Governor Brady was a former missionary, as was Loyal Lincoln Wirt, there is little doubt they were friends. But because his book was published thirty years after the fact, we doubt the exact conversation took place. Newspaper accounts from that time corroborate most of the events described in his book.

16 **"It's all a lie!"**: Wirt, *Alaskan Adventures*, 21.

16 **"It seemed as if a great albatross"**: Ibid., 19

17 **Gold dust was used as money**: Terrence Cole, *Banking on Alaska: The Story of the National Bank of Alaska*, 2 vols. (Anchorage: National Bank of Alaska, 2000), 1:15.

18 **"To those who contemplate"**: L. H. French, *Nome Nugget: Some of the Experiences of a Party of Gold Seekers in Northwestern Alaska in 1900* (Anchorage: Alaska Northwest Publishing Co., 1883).

19 **the U.S. Army Signal Corps**: David Marshall, "The Building of Alaska's Communication System," in Max L. Marshall, ed., *The Story of the U.S. Army Signal Corps* (New York: Franklin Watts, 1965).

20 **"if you didn't own a dog team"**: Former deputy U.S. Marshal Hansen as told to the Edingtons, *Tundra, Romance and Adventure on Alaskan Trails* (New York & London: Century Company, 1930; hereafter cited as Hansen, *Tundra*), 69.

20 **"It was said at the time"**: Lorna Coppinger, *The World of Sled Dogs* (New York: Howell Book House, 1977), 42.

21 **"gentle anything on four legs"**: Barrett Willoughby, *Gentlemen Unafraid* (New York & London: G. P. Putnams Sons, 1928), 142.

22 **"Is Alaska a dog country"**: Jack Hines, "This Aims to Be Dog Country," *Everybody's Magazine* (n.d.), Wickersham Collection, Rasmuson.

22 **sweepstakes trail**: Esther Birdsall Darling, *The Great Dog Races of Nome, Official Souvenir History* (Nome: 1916); also Allan, *Gold*. Darling often sponsored Allan in the sweepstakes.

23 **"GONE TO THE DOGS"**: Willoughby, *Gentlemen Unafraid*, 96. Willoughby (along with Darling, Allan, and a number of other residents in Nome) described the carnival atmosphere in Nome during the sweepstakes.

24 **"more like dealing on the stock exchange"**: Ibid.

25 **his "K9 Corps"**: Coppinger, *The World of Sled Dogs*, 68. Scotty Allan also recalled in his biography the details of recruiting sled dogs to serve the French army during World War I.

26 **"It was enough to make one forget"**: Allan, *Gold*, 269.

26 **Since about 60 percent of Alaskan society:** Cole, *Banking on Alaska*, 84.

26 **Nome breakdown of population:** Kenneth A. Ungermann breaks down the population in Nome for 1925 between whites and Eskimos in *The Race to Nome* (New York: Harper & Row, 1963), which has since been accepted. Newspapers at the time refer only to a population of "more than a thousand."

27 **"places seemed to straighten up":** Dufresne, *My Way*, 13.

27 **huge, electric-powered dredges:** Doug Beckstead, *What Is a Dredge*, April 9, 2001, www.nps.gov/yuch/Expanded/mining_history/coal_creek /what_is_a_dredge.htm (January 2002). Beckstead, a historian, wrote about the types of dredges used in Alaska and the Yukon Territory.

27 **"like last year's bird nest":** Summers-Wolf correspondence.

28 **"It was so big and bright":** Lula Welch, "Northland Doctor's Wife."

28 **"If there happened to be":** Curtis Welch, "An Unfinished Memoir," 5.

28 **"a hall as run-down as its old movies":** Dufresne, *My Way*, 30.

29 **The houses were built about two-thirds:** John Poling, *A History of the Nome, Alaska Public Schools: 1899 to 1958; From the Gold Rush to Statehood*, master's thesis, University of Alaska, 1970. Poling was a former resident of Nome. His thesis describes the social life in Nome as well as the integration of the Eskimos into the community.

29 **Walsh owned the only two cows:** Drawn from interviews with former Nome resident Joe Walsh in 2001 while he was a resident at the Pioneer Home in Fairbanks, Alaska. Sadly, Joe Walsh has since passed away.

Chapter Two: Outbreak

33 **Welch's medical routine:** Lula Welch, "Northland Doctor's Wife"; Curtis Welch, "An Unfinished Memoir."

33 **Margaret Solvey Eide:** Welch Report. Welch does not name Eide in his report, but the details of her illness correspond with reports in the *Nome Nugget* and her death certificate, filled out by Welch the day after her death.

34 **"asparkle with tinsel":** Recollections of Christmas in Nome are drawn from Jim Walsh, one of the ten children of the pioneer Walsh family whose history paralleled Nome's.

35 **"the whole town was alive":** The tradition of Community Christmas was inaugurated in Nome in the mid-1920s and recalled in colorful

detail by a Nome historian and early resident, Carrie McLain, in a Christmas edition of the *Nome Nugget* (December 24, 1966).

36 **"Death from tonsillitis is rare":** Welch Report.

36 **deaths of unnamed Natives:** Nome's Centennial Cemetery Project under Cussy Kauer's direction aided us in reconstructing the onset of the epidemic from the death certificates. Databases of deaths in Nome by date and victim, as well as Kaver's burial records and restoration of grave markers in Nome's cemeteries, all helped to fill out the sequence of events missing from newspaper accounts and Welch's medical report, though the records are incomplete and in some cases contradictory.

36 **Billy Barnett's symptoms and treatment:** Welch Report. Welch does not name Barnett, but the length of the boy's stay in hospital and his symptoms correspond closely with reports in the *Nome Nugget.*

36 **"anxious, struggling, pitiful expression":** H. K. Mulford Co., *The Present Status of Diphtheria Antitoxic Serum* (Philadelphia & Chicago: H. K. Mulford, 1897 or 1898), 17. The book reprints the writings of several doctors. This quote is from Lester Keller, M.D., writing in *Medical World* (November 1896), Merck Archives, Merck & Co.

37 **"The most distressing":** Evelynn Maxine Hammonds, "The Search for Perfect Control: A Social History of Diphtheria, 1880–1930," Harvard University, 1993, 24. Hammonds quotes from the work of Dr. Victor C. Vaughan, *Epidemiology and Public Health*, (St. Louis: C. V. Mosby Co., 1922), 3.

37 **"I didn't feel justified":** Welch Report.

37 **might send the community:** Welch Report.

39 **"In several cases":** Mulford Co., *The Present Status of Diphtheria*, 17. Lester Keller, M.D.

39 **"I hardly feel competent":** Welch to Cumming, June 18, 1925, National Archives.

39 **fears that the disease would destroy the colonies:** Ernest Caulfield, M.D., "A True History of the Terrible Epidemic Vulgarly Called the Throat Distemper which occurred in His Majesty's New England Colonies between the years 1735–1740," *Yale Journal of Biology and Medicine* (1935), 2.

40 **"the woeful effects of Original Sin":** Ibid., 22.

40 **"It frequently begins":** W. Barry Wood, Jr., *Miasmas and Molecules* (New York & London: Columbia University Press, 1961), 2.

40 **"All that I have seen":** Ibid., 4.

41 **"You have done all the good":** Allan Chase, *Magic Shots* (New York: William Morrow, 1982), 168.

42 **Welch also realized that the disease could move:** Welch sent several telegrams to Washington expressing his concern that the epidemic could spread beyond Nome.

42 **"The Natives showed absolutely":** Governor Riggs in his annual report to the Secretary of the Interior, *Reports of the Department of the Interior,* vol. 2 (1919), National Archives, RG 348.

43 **Welch was shaken from his troubled sleep:** Welch Report, February 16, 1925.

43 **the "strong, elemental" nature:** *Hartford Courant,* February 7, 1925.

43 **"one mass of fetid, stinking":** Welch Report, February 16.

44 **regain his professional composure:** Lula Welch, "Northland Doctor's Wife."

Chapter Three: Quarantine

47 **comfortable office and the council meeting:** Phoebe West, "I Remember Nome," *Alaska Sportsman* (April 1962); "Nomeites Concerned," *Nome Nugget,* January 24, 1925; Welch Report; Ungermann, *Race to Nome,* 17–21.

48 **Bessie Stanley's treatment:** Welch Report.

49 **"It was impossible to get anyone":** Written in a letter dated February 9, 1919, immediately after influenza tore through Nome. Author unknown (Carrie McLain Memorial Museum, Nome).

49 **"Natives dying every few minutes":** From the flurry of telegrams sent from Mayor Lomen to Governor Riggs, Department of the Interior officials, and Bureau of Education members responsible for the welfare of Natives in Nome. "Not a single Eskimo escaped influenza infection" . . . "Eskimos dying like rats" . . . "Render all relief possible," were among the urgent telegrams found in the Records of the Department of the Interior (Governor's Correspondence, National Archives, RG 348).

50 **"Were it within your power":** In a letter Father Lafortune wrote to his sister on December 8, 1918, quoted in Father Louis Renner's biography of the brave missionary who devoted more than sixty years to the Eskimos of Seward Peninsula, *Pioneer Missionary.* Louis Renner, S.J., *Pioneer Missionary to the Bering Strait Eskimos: Bellarmine Lafortune, S.J.* (Portland, OR: Binford & Mort, 1979).

50 **"mowed down like grass":** Entry in Father Lafortune's House Diary written at the end of 1918, quoted in Renner's biography.

51 Welch suggested that every school: Welch Report; *Nome Nugget*, January 24, 1925.

51 one was to be coded for all points in Alaska: Ungermann, *Race to Nome*, 20.

51 "An epidemic of diphtheria": Welch bulletin to Cumming, January 22, 1925, National Archives.

52 Walshes . . . Jean Summers-Wolf remembered: Summers-Wolf correspondence; authors' interview with Joe Walsh.

52 "An epidemic of diphtheria": "Nomeites Concerned," *Nome Nugget*, January 24, 1925.

52 Dora and Mary Stanley: Welch Report; Daily Medical Reports, Carrie McLain Memorial Museum archives (hereafter cited as Medical Reports).

53 Rynning family: Medical Reports.

53 "My nurses are the only consultants": Welch Report.

54 "we had plenty of doctors and hospitals": Charlotte Offen, "Angel of the Yukon," *True West* (March–April 1974).

54 Morgan's visits to Sandspit and ensuing dialogue: Ibid. Morgan was assigned to Nome to take over duties from Bertha Seville, who was an active Registered Nurse in Nome since 1917 until 1925.

55 they had about twenty confirmed cases: Medical Reports.

56 to travel the 674 miles: Early records citing the distance of the mail trail vary: 674 is the generally accepted figure. These trails in Alaska are not permanent, and maintaining them is a continual fight against nature. Encroaching rivers and erosion continually take away and add miles to an impermanent route. Bends in the Tanana River, for instance, have moved a distance of over five miles in this past century alone.

56 Mark Summers had a plan: Summers-Wolf correspondence. Mark Summers's daughter also recalls the relationship her father and family had with the Seppalas.

56 "King of the Trail": The term appears to have been used first in reference to Alaska's ever important mail drivers. With the advent of dog racing on those same working trails, Seppala was anointed "King of the Trail." Correspondence and telegrams from the driver himself show he often signed himself thus.

56 The mayor had long been an advocate: "Nomeites Concerned," *Nome Nugget*, January 24, 1925.

57 "Serious epidemic of diphtheria": Maynard to Sutherland, January 23, 1925, reprinted in "Telegraphic," *Nome Nugget*, January 31, 1925.

59 **Leonhard Seppala—personal details:** Elizabeth Ricker with Leonhard Seppala, *Seppala: Alaskan Dog Driver* (Boston: Little, Brown, 1930); Raymond Thompson, *Seppala's Saga of the Sled Dog*, 2 vols. (Lynnwood, WA: 1977); and Ungermann's *Race to Nome*.

60 **He was something of a show-off:** Author's interview with Joe Walsh.

60 **So much was at stake:** Leonhard Seppala, interview by the *Boston Herald*, February 20, 1927, Leonhard Seppala Collection, Rasmuson.

61 **"The dogs always came first":** Charlotte Widrig, "The Golden Days of Dog-Sled Racing," *Seattle Times*, March 28, 1954.

63 **"The birchwood runners of my sled":** Leonhard Seppala, with Raymond Thompson, "I Met My First Dog Team 60 Years Ago," *Alaska Sportsman* (May 1961).

63 **"Every time the telephone rang":** Ricker, *Alaskan Dog Driver*, 290.

64 **"like a reindeer":** Authors' interview with Joe Walsh.

65 **"a piece of blubber":** Waldemar Bogoras, *The Chukchee*, Publications of the Jesup North Pacific Expedition, vol. 7, 1904–09, American Museum of Natural History Research Library. Bogoras provides one of the more reliable accounts of the dogs of Siberia.

66 **William Goosak heard about dogs:** Coppinger, *World of Sled Dogs*, 86.

66 **"Siberian rats":** Nome residents at the time also referred to the Siberians as "fuzzy wuzzy lap dogs" or simply as "rats." See also John Douglas Tanner, Jr., *Alaska Trails—Siberian Dogs* (Wheat Ridge, CO: Hoflin Publishing, 1986), and Ungermann, *Race to Nome*, 59.

67 **would have broken the bank in Nome:** Earl and Natalie Norris, "A Short Alaskan History of the Siberian Husky," in Pamela Thomas, Ann Stead, and Nancy Wolfe, eds., *The Siberian Husky* 3rd edn. (Elkhorn, WI: International Siberian Husky Club, 1994), 42.

67 **"howling from every porthole":** Tanner, *Alaska Trails*, 18.

67 **"I did not win the race":** O. A. Braafladt, "Men of Iron, Dogs of Speed," *Alaska Sportsman* (December 1937).

67 **"There seems to be almost no limit":** Letter by Seppala, Seppala Archives, International Siberian Husky Club, Wisconsin.

68 **"I literally fell in love with them":** Leonhard Seppala, with Raymond Thompson, "Nome Dog Races," *Alaska Sportsman* (July 1961).

68 **or "raving mad":** Willoughby, *Gentlemen Unafraid*, 85.

68 **"It was truly a land":** Seppala, "Nome Dog Races," *Alaska Sportsman* (July 1961).

68 **dispatches from the racecourse:** Reprinted in Allan, *Gold*, 209.

69 **"They told me I came in":** Ibid., 217.

70 **He felt nervous and excited:** Seppala, "Nome Dog Races," *Alaska Sportsman*. (July 1961).

70 **"By the time we were making":** Ibid.

70 **"the more I thought it over the less":** Ricker, *Alaskan Dog Driver,* 209. An in-depth description of Seppala's first sweepstake race also appears in Seppala, "Nome Dog Races," and Thompson's *Seppala's Saga.*

70 **"I don't know what":** "Renowned Dog Musher of All Alaska Sweepstake Races Talks at College," *Farthest-North Collegian,* December 1, 1933.

71 **"their simple, canine faith":** Thompson, *Seppala's Saga,* 1:49.

71 **"I felt like a loaded gun":** Leonhard Seppala, with Raymond Thompson, "I Won the Nome Sweepstakes," *Alaska Sportsman* (November 1961).

72 **"smiled back at me enigmatically":** Ricker, *Alaskan Dog Driver,* 219.

72 **"could see a team way back":** Ibid., 220.

73 **"Seppala's team is all in":** Ibid., 223.

74 **"They were dragging along slowly":** Ibid., 224.

75 **"Scotty came dashing after me":** Ibid., 229.

75 **"That man is super-human":** "Seppala Triumph Attributed to Hypnotism; Just 'Clucked' and His Dogs Raced to Victory," *The New York Times,* February 14, 1927. The competitor's name has been reported as Si Mason or Hiram Mason of New Hampshire.

76 **"I am proud of my racing trophies":** Seppala Archives, International Siberian Husky Club.

76 **"inseparably linked":** Foreword by Frank Dufresne, letter dated February 15, 1927, in Elizabeth Ricker, *Togo's Fireside Reflections* (Lewiston, ME: Lewiston Journal Printshop, 1928).

76 **"Go to it":** Ibid.

76 **"with a sense of security":** Ricker, *Alaskan Dog Driver,* 280.

Chapter Five: Flying Machines

79 **"Could aviator at Fairbanks put plane":** Sutherland to Thompson, January 26, 1925, reprinted in *Fairbanks Daily News-Miner,* same date. This issue of the *News-Miner* also gives a full account of Thompson's actions that morning, as well as those of the mechanic and Roy Darling.

80 keep up their **"flattened spirits":** Mary Lee Cadwell Davis, *We Are All Alaskans* (Boston: W. A. Wilde Co., 1931), 132.

80 **"Lost His Chocolate Drop":** Ibid., 153. Also quoted as "Lost His Little Chocolate Drop."

81 **"drinking homebrew":** Jean Clark Potter, *The Flying North* (New York: Macmillan, 1947), 37. Potter writes in depth about Fairbanks in the 1920s and the first Alaskan bush pilots. Her work includes the role W. F. Thompson played in starting an aviation company in the town.

82 **"crossroads city of the world":** Ibid., 35.

83 **"to try it on for size":** Robert Stevens, *Alaskan Aviation History*, 2 vols. (Des Moines, WA: Polynyas Press, 1990), 1:37.

84 **"cheerful, forceful, active":** Military Records of Roy Andrew Darling, National Archives, RG 125, Records of the Judge Advocate General of the Navy, Navy Examining Boards 1890–1941. The records also describe Darling's injuries.

84 the **"broken flyer":** *Fairbanks Daily News-Miner*, January 26, 1925.

85 **"had to go hanging onto the tail":** Ibid.

86 **"hit the air for Nome, rain or shine":** Ibid.

86 **"The atmosphere is not right":** Ibid.

87 **"be of good cheer":** Thompson to *Nome Nugget*, January 26, 1925, reprinted in "Telegraphic," *Nome Nugget*, January 31, 1925.

87 **"I am allowing the dust of Washington":** *Fairbanks Daily News-Miner*, July 28, 1924.

88 **"Health Department will take":** Sutherland to Maynard, January 26, 1925, "Telegraphic," *Nome Nugget*, January 31, 1925.

89 **Beeson was a competent:** Paul Beeson, "Rushing the Serum to the Rescue: A Long House Call," *Resident & Staff Physician* (April 1990).

90 the **conductor, Frank Knight:** Ungermann, *Race to Nome*, 52–53.

90 **"Appreciate your prompt action":** Bone to Beeson, January 27, 1925, Telegram, National Archives.

90 **governor had a kind and warm way about him:** *Baltimore Sun*, August 1, 1923.

92 **"unfit for habitation":** E. A. Steece, Supervising Architect, Treasury Department to Washington, Report, July 7, 1924, Alaska State Archives, Territorial Governor's Office, General Correspondence.

92 **"It will not be long":** Claus-M. Naske, *An Interpretative History of Alaska Statehood* (Anchorage: Alaska Northwest Publishing Co., 1973), 49.

92 **"interlocked, overlapped, cumbersome":** Scott C. Bone, "Alaska from the Inside," *Saturday Evening Post*, August 8, 1925, Daniel Sutherland Papers, Rasmuson. In his article, Bone was reiterating the words of former Secretary of Interior Franklin K. Lane.

92 **maimed the pioneer spirit:** Scott C. Bone, "Alaska—Last of American Frontiers," *Elks Magazine* (July 1922), Daniel Sutherland Papers, Rasmuson.

92 **"No one understands Alaska":** Scott C. Bone, "The Land That Uncle Sam Bought and Then Forgot," *Review of Reviews* (April 1922), Daniel Sutherland Papers, Rasmuson.

92 **the serum could get bogged down:** Bone, "Alaska from the Inside," *Saturday Evening Post*, August 8, 1925.

94 **"an almost continuous succession":** "Admiral Watson Here After One Stormy Voyage," *Alaska Daily Empire*, January 26, 1925. The paper also gives specifics about the cold weather in the Interior.

94 **"shaken up by the rough passage":** Ibid.

94 **"rolled like an old-fashioned":** Phoebe West, "I Remember Nome," *Alaska Sportsman* (April 1962).

95 **it "came within the rays of the bonfire":** Potter, *Flying North*, 41. Details of Eielson's flight appear in the pilot's report, sent to the Second Assistant Postmaster General, Colonel Paul Henderson of the U.S. Post Office in charge of the Air Mail Service, William Mitchell Papers, microfilm, Rasmuson Library. See also Carl Benjamin Eielson, "Aeroplaning in Alaska," Daniel Sutherland Papers, Rasmuson.

95 **"We found him grinning":** Barrett Willoughby, *Alaskans All* (Boston & New York: Houghton Mifflin, 1933), 107.

96 **President Calvin Coolidge:** "Eielson Tells of His Experience," *Alaska Weekly*, April 11, 1924.

96 **"There are many things which must":** Potter, *Flying North*, 43.

96 **"lighthouses in the sky":** Cecil Roseberry, *The Challenging Skies* (Garden City, NY: Doubleday & Co., 1966), 35.

97 **Wien "jumped off":** Potter, *Flying North*, 122.

98 **"flying inside a milk bottle":** Ibid., 66. The pilot was Joe Crosson.

98 **"Airplanes can't fly into 60 mph winds":** Ira Harkey, "Pioneer Bush Pilot: The Story of Noel Wien," *Alaska Magazine*, part 2 (December 1975). Excerpted from Harkey, *Pioneer Bush Pilot: The Story of Noel Wien* (Seattle: University of Washington Press, 1974).

98 **number of forced landings dropped:** Herschel Smith, *A History of Aircraft Piston Engines* (Manhattan, KS: Sunflower University Press, 1986).

99 **"reconnoitered and explored":** Roseberry, *Challenging Skies*, 281.

100 **In his opinion, the equipment was inadequate:** Bone's concerns about a flight are evident in several of the telegrams he wrote to Washington.

101 **"Nature has many tricks":** Jack London, "The White Silence," *Northland Stories* (New York: Penguin Books, 1997), 3.

102 **"To see the excitement":** Gold Rush Centennial Task Force, State of

Alaska, "Gold Rush Stories: The Mail Must Go Through," 1999; www.library.state.ak.us/goldrush/stories/mail.htm (March 2001).

103 **"You'd have to be on time":** Pete Curran, Jr., interview by Tom Beck, transcript 4, August 1980, Iditarod Trail Project Oral History Program, Bureau of Land Management, Rasmuson.

103 **"There were days the poor dogs":** Bill McCarty, interview by Tom Beck, transcript 13, September 1980, ibid. The quotation appears in the transcript as: "I remember the days the poor dogs, they hated to go, going against—up river against the head wind, cold. I had to work on dogs' feet, putting moccasins on dogs. When it was that cold, 50 or 60 below . . . they didn't like it."

104 **"Them feet and me are goin' ":** Sherry Simpson, "Heroes of the Mail Trail," *Alaska Magazine* (February 1996).

105 **"I called to the man":** William Mitchell, *The Opening of Alaska: 1901–1903*, William Mitchell Papers, microfilm, 45, Rasmuson.

105 **"Please engage relay dog teams":** Bone to Wetzler, January 26, 1925, National Archives.

106 **"Inspector Wetzler instructed":** Bone to Welch, January 26, 1925, National Archives.

106 **to seeing "the big city":** Yukon-Koyukuk School District of Alaska, *Edgar Kallands: A Biography* (Fairbanks: Spirit Mountain Press, 1982), 45. There has been some question as to which town Kallands transported the serum. Some early accounts put his relay leg from Nine Mile Cabin to Kokrines. However, in his biography Kallands said he took the serum from Shannon and traveled to Manley Hot Springs. Several newspaper accounts at the time also reported that Kallands traveled between Tolovana and Manley.

106 **Harry Pitka:** Ungermann, *Race to Nome*, 76. Ungermann provides a list of the serum run drivers, as do several telegrams in the National Archives.

107 **"Governor Bone has evidently":** *Fairbanks Daily News-Miner,* January 27, 1925.

107 **"Woe unto the public official":** "William Forepaugh," manuscript, n.d., John Clark Collection, Rasmuson.

107 **"Fairbanks could help Nome":** *Fairbanks Daily News-Miner*, January 28, 1925.

Chapter Six: Hunters of the North

This chapter was partly inspired by the many works of two of the great arctic anthropologists, Vilhjalmur Stefansson and Richard K. Nelson. Of particular interest were Stefansson's *The Friendly Arctic* (New York: Macmillan, 1943) and *Hunters of the Great North* (New York: Harcourt, Brace & Company, 1922); and Nelson's *Hunters of the Northern Forest* (Chicago and London: University of Chicago Press, 1973) and *Hunters of the Northern Ice* (Chicago & London: University of Chicago Press, 1969).

Private letters and unpublished manuscripts of missionaries from the 1900s whose lives were devoted to the Natives of Alaska, most notably Father Lafortune in service of the Eskimos of Seward Peninsula and Father Jette in service of the Athabaskans of the Interior were invaluable (Alaska Mission Collection, UAF).

The Smithsonian ethnologist Edward William Nelson, in his study, *Eskimos About Bering Strait* (Washington: Smithsonian Institution Press, 1983, first published 1899), provides an invaluable inventory of their material culture. *Crossroads of Continents: Cultures of Siberia and Alaska*, ed. William W. Fitzhugh and Aron Cromwell (Washington, D.C., & London: Smithsonian Institution Press, 1988), was also useful, particularly the essays on "Maritime Economies of the North Pacific Rim" by Jean-Loup Rousselot, William W. Fitzhugh, and Aron Cromwell, and "Needles and Animals: Women's Magic" by Valerie Chaussonnet.

Anthropologist Wendell H. Oswalt's fascinating *Eskimos and Explorers* (Nebraska: University of Nebraska Press, 1999) paints a cultural portrait of the Eskimos at the moment of contact with Europeans; Dorothy Jean Ray's portrait of Eskimos of the Bering Strait region right up to the most cataclysmic impact of them all, the 1900 discovery of gold in Nome, helped fill in the picture. Articles published in the journal *Arctic Anthropology*, and the many histories of dogs and their evolution—as well as continuing research on the subject by academics on the Internet—helped to trace the evidence of dog traction and the earliest uses of dog sledding.

Chapter Seven: The "Rule of the 40s"

137 just shy of 9:00 P.M.: Wetzler to Bone, January 27, 1925, Telegram, National Archives. The telegram puts Shannon's departure time from Nenana at 9:00 P.M.

138 details on Shannon before the run: Churchill Fisher, "Healy Storekeeper," *Alaska Sportsman* (November 1942); Bill Shannon, interview by *Seward Daily Gateway*, March 7, 1925; Shannon interview by *Tacoma News Tribune*, n.d., Seppala Collection, Rasmuson; Ungermann, *Race to Nome*, 60–62.

139 the "rule of the 40s": Will Forsberg, "Keeping Your Dogs Healthy in Cold Weather," *Mushing Magazine* (January–February 1997).

139 "Traveling at 50 below": Hudson Stuck, *Ten Thousand Miles with a Dog Sled: A Narrative of Winter Travel in Interior Alaska* (Lincoln & London: University of Nebraska Press, 1988), 14.

140 "a lost glove means a lost hand": E. D. Stokes, "The Race for Life," *Public Health Reports* (May–June 1996).

141 "a sound as of someone pounding": Hansen, *Tundra*, 138.

143 "Hell, Wetz": Bill Shannon, interview by *Tacoma News Tribune*, n.d., Seppala Collection, Rasmuson. In his interviews with the press, Shannon spoke in detail about his run, providing details on the weather and the trail as well his and the dogs' condition.

145 "[They] broke through every step": Scott, *Tracks Across Alaska* (New York: Atlantic Monthly Press, 1990), 96.

146 "A man is only as good as his dogs": Hansen, *Tundra*, 93–94.

146 a "crystalline tomb": Ibid. Hansen describes his drum ice story on pp. 108–11.

148 "large enough to drag down": Bill Shannon, interview by *Minneapolis Star Daily*, May 18, 1925.

148 his attempts to get blood: *Tacoma News Tribune*, n.d.

149 "fairly stupefied by the cold": Shannon interviewed by *Seward Daily Gateway*. Shannon's attempts to stay warm and his comment about being stupefied by the cold indicate the severity of his hypothermia.

150 "long conscious fight": Stuck, *Ten Thousand Miles*, 68.

150 "All of us who have traveled": Ibid.

150 arrival at Minto, coffee, condition of Shannon and dogs: Shannon interviews by *Seward Daily Gateway*; *Tacoma News Tribune*, n.d.; and unidentified newspaper, Seppala Collection, Rasmuson.

Chapter Eight: Along the Yukon River

153 dangling the container from the rafters: Shannon interview by *Seward Daily Gateway*.

153 The cabin was probably no warmer: Although Shannon noted the temperature outdoors, he never noted it inside the cabin. The temperature varied in a roadhouse: it was always pretty warm by the stove because drying out equipment and clothes was considered an essential service, but usually pretty cool where the bunks were located.

154 **"lung scorching" . . . leaving dogs behind:** Shannon interview by *Seward Daily Gateway*.

154 **Seppala's pre-run preparations:** Ricker, *Alaskan Dog Driver*, 289–91; Thompson, *Seppala's Saga*, 2:24–25; Ungermann, *Race to Nome*, 64–66.

155 **uproar in kennel, cheering crowd:** Ricker, *Alaskan Dog Driver*, 291; Thompson, *Seppala's Saga*, 2:25.

156 **other patient histories:** Medical Reports. The reports note the patients' symptoms and indicate who received serum.

157 **would not wear off:** Thompson, *Seppala's Saga*, 2:25.

158 **Summers had warned Seppala:** Seppala wrote often that Summers had warned him against crossing the sea ice.

158 **"It is absolutely almost impossible":** Olaf Swenson, *Northwest of the World; Forty Years Trading and Hunting in Northern Siberia* (New York: Dodd, Mead & Co., 1944), 182–83.

160 **Togo's early history:** Ricker, *Alaskan Dog Driver*, 283–87; Thompson, *Seppala's Saga*, 2:14–16; Ungermann, *Race to Nome*, 113–18, and Togo's own "biography," Ricker's *Togo's Fireside Reflections*, and *The New York Times Magazine*, January 5, 1930. All these works give extensive details about Togo's life and early experiences on the trail.

160 **"showing all the signs":** Ungermann, *Race to Nome*, 115.

160 **"A dog so devoted to":** Thompson, *Seppala's Saga*, 2:14.

161 **"Like a lot of humans":** Ibid., 15.

161 **"squealing like a little pig":** Ricker, *Alaskan Dog Driver*, 285.

162 **an "infant prodigy":** Ibid., 287.

162 **"Steady, Hurricane":** The account that follows is drawn from Elsie Noble Caldwell, *Alaska Trail Dogs* (New York: R. R. Smith, 1945), 116–17. Caldwell's work has an amazing array of lead dog stories.

164 **"crossed the ice on the big crack":** Willoughby, *Gentlemen Unafraid*, 161.

164 **"You can't tell me that a dog":** Ibid., 162.

165 **"pretending indifference":** John O'Brien, *By Dog Sled for Byrd; 1600 Miles Across Antarctic Sea Ice* (Chicago: Thomas S. Rockwell Co., 1931), 180. Colonel Norman D. Vaughan continued to drive dogs after the expedition and became an active member of the mushing community and the author of *My Life of Adventure* and *With Byrd at the Bottom of the World*.

165 **"Thus completely foiled in this":** Edgerton Young, *My Dogs in the Northland* (London: S. W. Partridge & Co., 1902), 170.

166 **"He was my dog":** *Edgar Kallands,* 14.

166 **". . . when I go away and come back":** Ibid., 50.

167 **"I want you to go back":** Ibid., 45.

167 **"It was 56 below, but I didn't notice":** Bill Sherwonit, *Iditarod: The Great Race to Nome* (Anchorage: Northwest Books, 1991), 35.

168 **"Antitoxin departed Tolovana":** Wetzler to Bone, January 28, 1925, National Archives.

168 **would be weeks before he would once again:** Unidentified newspaper, Seppala Collection, Rasmuson.

168 **"What those dogs did":** *Tacoma News Tribune,* n.d.

168 **"If ever their master comes":** Ann Mariah Cook, *Running North: A Yukon Adventure* (Chapel Hill, NC: Algonquin Books of Chapel Hill, 1998), 98.

Chapter Nine: Red Tape

171 **Usually at this time:** West, "I Remember Nome," *Alaska Sportsman* (April 1962).

171 **yet by that evening:** Various newspaper reports and telegrams indicate that town officials had thought, or at least hoped, that the epidemic had been contained.

171 **Daniel Kialook:** Medical Reports.

172 **Even without Schick Tests:** Welch requested Schick Tests in his telegrams to Washington.

173 **"The situation is bad":** Contents of telegram printed in "Authorizes Flier to Make Nome Dash," *The New York Times,* January 31, 1925.

173 **This third batch:** A "third batch" of serum is referred to in several telegrams sent between Nome and Nenana and Juneau on January 28, 1925, January 29, 1925, and February 4, 1925.

174 **"I am a physician":** Welch to Public Health Service, January 21, 1925, National Archives, RG 90.

175 **"who suffered for the sufferers":** Bone to C. R. Hope, Universal News Service, article, January 30, 1925, National Archives, RG 90.

176 **In 1922, some 60,000 households:** Robert Hughes, "Passion for the New," *Time* magazine, March 9, 1998.

177 **". . . It is an unpeopled country":** Scott C. Bone, Annual Report, 1924, microfilm, Rasmuson.

177 **"Help immediately!":** Associated Press, January 30, 1925. The plea appeared in several newspapers.

178 **"There is no denying":** Editorial, *Alaska Daily Empire*, February 3, 1925.

178 **"Epidemic Grows Graver":** *The Washington Post*, January 31, 1925.

179 **"the greatest humanitarian service":** *The New York Sun*, January 30, 1925.

179 **"Aviator Darling of Fairbanks":** Sutherland to Maynard, January 29, 1925, "Telegraphic," *Nome Nugget*, January 31, 1925.

181 **"Even so, the flight":** *Seattle Union Record*, January 30, 1925.

181 **"would take longer":** Ibid.

182 a **"cruiser carrying airplane":** Loring Pickering to Surgeon General Cumming, January 30, 1925, National Archives, RG 90.

182 **"not permit this epidemic":** Ibid.

183 **"We have been conferring":** "Navy Officials to Rely on Dog Teams for Rescue," *The New York World*, February 1, 1925. The story was written on January 31.

184 **"from what I know":** *Seattle Times*, January 31, 1925.

184 **". . . suggest aviator Darling":** Sutherland to Thompson, January 30, 1925, reprinted in *Fairbanks Daily News-Miner*, January 31, 1925.

185 **"use his discretion":** Acting Surgeon General to Bone, January 30, 1925, National Archives.

185 **"Nome looks to Fairbanks":** *Fairbanks Daily News-Miner*, January 30, 1925.

187 to **"spare no expense":** Summers to Traeger, January 30, 1925 (contents of message printed in the *Nome Nugget*, January 31, 1925). Some sources report that Nome's health board initially made the decision to speed up the relay. We believe it was Governor Bone, who was the ultimate authority in Alaska on the rescue mission.

188 **gloved hands froze to the sled's:** Associated Press, January 29, 1925.

188 **details on Charlie Evans's run:** Jeffrey Richardson, "Serum Runner Remembers," *Senior Voice* (1986); Charlie Evans, interview by Tom Beck, transcript, September 12, 1980, Iditarod Trail Project Oral History Program, Bureau of Land Management, Rasmuson; Matthew Donohue, "All in a Day's Work: Mushers Recall Serum Run of 1925," *Alaska Magazine* (March 1980); Ungermann, *Race to Nome*, 80–82; and Don Bowers, *Iditarod Trail Notes 2000*, Iditarod Trail Sled Dog Race, www.iditarod.com (August 2000).

190 **"It would come over me":** Hansen, *Tundra*, 282.

190 **"let the dogs go":** Richardson, "Serum Runner Remembers."

191 **"I can't stop":** Ibid.

191 **he moved to the front of the team:** Coppinger, *World of Sled Dogs*, 63.

192 **"It was real cold":** Ibid.

192 **the "big animal":** Sidney Huntington, as told to Jim Rearden, *Shadows on the Koyukuk* (Portland, OR: Alaska Northwest Books, 1993), 172. Huntington describes the bear hunt in these memoirs of living along the Koyukuk River in Alaska's Interior.

Chapter Ten: The Ice Factory

195 **"the ice factory":** William Stringer, Professor Emeritus, University of Alaska, Fairbanks, Dept. of Geology and Geophysics, interview by the authors at Fairbanks, August 2000.

199 **Gonangnan run:** Ungermann, *Race to Nome*, 106–10. Ungermann is the main source for Gonangnan's experience on the trail. The driver left little record of his trip. Detail on the trail comes from Don Bowers's *Iditarod Trail Notes 2000*, www.iditarod.com (August 2000), and his book *Back of the Pack: An Iditarod Rookie Musher's Alaska Pilgrimage to Nome* (Anchorage: Publication Consultants, 1998), 334–35.

199 **Over the past few days:** The wind direction is based on anecdotal accounts. These accounts contradict weather maps of the time, which are not fully reliable. Both the anecdotal accounts and the weather maps, however, confirm that on the day of Gonangnan and Seppala's run, the wind was blowing offshore. Given the wind's strength, the ice would have been under threat of breaking up with or without the past few days of an onshore breeze.

203 **"blowing so hard":** Ungermann, *Race to Nome*, 107.

203 **"the edge of the planet":** Bowers, *Iditarod Trail Notes 2000*, www.iditarod.com (August 2000). The Web site is a comprehensive source for further information on the Iditarod and its participants.

204 **the whiteout conditions cleared:** It is not exactly clear at what point the whiteout conditions cleared. Most likely Gonangnan regained reference points when he reached Norton Sound.

204 **at gale force, about 40 miles per hour:** This is an estimated wind speed based upon the prevailing wind conditions along this stretch of coast, anecdotal accounts by other drivers, and the strength of the storm brewing to the south. The drivers referred to gale-force winds, which are between 39 and 54 mph. The storm, which had not reached its height during Gonangnan's run, was packing winds in excess of 55 mph, accord-

ing to weather maps of 1925. These are located at University of Alaska, Fairbanks, Geophysical Institute.

205 **"Would advise keeping all":** Welch to Bureau of Education, January 31, 1925, National Archives.

205 **"Nome Situation Critical":** *Seattle Post-Intelligencer,* February 1, 1925.

206 **". . . have received information":** Welch to Surgeon General, January 31, 1925, National Archives.

206 **The wind was behind him:** Leonhard Seppala, with Raymond Thompson, "When Nome Needed Serum," *Alaska Sportsman* (May 1961). Seppala describes his round-trip journey in detail.

207 ***"The serum! The serum! I have it here!":*** Ibid.

208 **had his own daughter to worry about:** The reports vary as to whether or not Sigrid contracted diphtheria. One account said she suffered a severe sore throat in late December, another that she contracted the disease during the epidemic. In an interview with the authors in early 2002, Sigrid said she did not catch diphtheria.

208 **"ready to bet their final ounce":** *Berkeley Gazette,* January 31, 1925, Seppala Collection, Rasmuson.

208 **"always argued that there's nothing":** Ibid.

208 **"There isn't any quit in him":** *San Francisco Bulletin,* January 31, 1925, Seppala Collection, Rasmuson.

209 **but drive as if he were in a race:** Ricker, *Alaskan Dog Driver,* 292.

210 **"Togo seemed to understand":** Leonhard Seppala, interview in *Boston Sunday Post,* January 27, 1927.

210 **"until it was twice looped":** Ibid.

211 **Occasionally, he leaned out:** Ungermann, *Race to Nome,* 123. Another technique Seppala may have used was to lay his hand on the ice and let it glide across the rough surface, on the alert for any vibration that would indicate ice was piling up or coming apart in the distance.

211 **fed them salmon and seal blubber:** Seppala, "Needed Serum," *Alaska Sportsman* (May 1961).

Chapter Eleven: Cold Glory

213 **"Maybe you go more closer":** Ricker, *Alaskan Dog Driver,* 293.

213 **details of Seppala's run:** Ricker, *Alaskan Dog Driver,* 293–94; Ungermann, *Race to Nome,* 129–31; Seppala, "Needed Serum," *Alaska Sportsman* (May 1961); Coppinger, *World of Sled Dogs,* 64. Detail on the trail comes from Bowers, *Iditarod Trail Notes* and *Back of the Pack,* 353.

215 **"even if the dogs manage":** *Seattle Star,* February 2, 1925.

216 **Mayor Maynard picked up the phone:** It was not fully clear who made the call to the roadhouse keeper in Solomon, but over the course of the epidemic Maynard became increasingly involved in the rescue mission. The call could also have been made by Summers, who was officially in charge of the relay in Nome.

217 **"Violent blizzard now on is delaying":** Welch to Bureau of Education, passed on to Public Health Service. The date of the message is unclear. It appears to have been sent on February 1. There is no doubt about the blizzard occurring on the date.

217 **in "constant motion from a heavy":** "Last Relay Driver Arrives at Nome with Serum," *Seattle Daily Times,* February 3, 1925.

218 **"Either you listened to him":** Jack Strege, Kaasen's great-nephew, interview by the authors, March 2002.

219 **"They couldn't have gone much":** Kasson (sic), *The World,* February 4, 1925.

220 **"I had seal mukluks":** Ibid.

220 **"We are up against it":** Stuck, *Ten Thousand Miles,* 104.

220 **"you don't know whether to pray":** Willoughby, *Gentlemen Unafraid,* 117.

221 **"air thick as smoke":** Ibid., 90.

221 **"sturdy and brave":** Ibid., 120–22.

223 **"Topkok is hell":** Kasson, *The World,* February 4, 1925.

223 **the course of the trail:** Bowers, *Back of Pack,* 360–61.

224 **"I didn't know where I was":** Kasson, *The World,* February 4, 1925.

224 **He patted the sled down:** Ibid.; Ungermann, *Race to Nome,* 152.

224 **"boosted" him along:** Kasson, *The World,* February 4, 1925.

225 **"Damn fine dog":** "Heroic Mushers Fasten Curb on Nome Epidemic," *The New York Sun,* February 4, 1925.

Chapter Twelve: Saved!

227 **The serum would have to be thawed:** Welch to Beeson, February 2, 1925, Telegram, National Archives.

227 **Welch went first:** Ibid.

228 **Margaret Curran's case:** "Disease Spreads in Nome," *Seattle Post-Intelligencer,* February 2, 1925.

229 **"I should feel much safer":** Welch to Beeson, February 2, 1925, Telegram, National Archives.

229 **a test drive down the main street:** *Fairbanks Daily News-Miner,* February 2, 1925.

229 **those who were seriously ill would recover:** Medical Reports.

229 **"I'm carrying on":** Unidentified newspaper, "Nome Correspondent, Stricken, Is on Job," February 4, 1925, dateline.

230 **"Six Dead As Plague Gains":** *San Francisco Chronicle,* February 5, 1925.

230 **"She was known to every sourdough":** "Nome Epidemic Is Checked," *Seattle Star,* February 5, 1925.

230 **"If this rate continues":** Sutherland to Bone, February 4, 1925, National Archives, RG 90.

231 **"This bureaucracy stands idly by":** *The Washington Post,* February 6, 1925.

231 **"Alarming reports sent":** "Governor Bone Takes Issue on Flight to Nome," *Alaska Daily Empire,* February 6, 1925.

231 **"as many spare engine parts":** North American Newspaper Alliance, carried in several newspapers, February 5, 1925.

232 **"It is most gallant of Darling":** "Serum to Be Taken by Plane," *Seattle Star,* February 3, 1925.

232 **officials in Nome were in "hysteria":** Bone to Wetzler, February 7, 1925. National Archives, RG 90.

233 **"solved between themselves":** "Darling Standing By with Mackie to Fly to Nome," *Anchorage Daily Alaskan,* February 3, 1925.

234 **"Our plane will pass the dogs":** "Airplane Hopes to Overtake Nome Dog Team Relay Today," *Seattle Daily Times,* February 9, 1925.

234 **would be "no great difficulty":** Darling to Bone, February 6, 1925, National Archives, RG 90.

235 **the number of recoveries was beginning:** It appears that Welch had first told DeVighne that the number of recoveries was beginning to outpace new cases in Nome on February 3 or 4, 1925.

236 **"We believe in the airship":** *Fairbanks Daily News-Miner,* February 10, 1925.

237 **"First Trip Air Mail Nome":** *Nome Nugget,* June 20, 1925.

238 **"Dilapidated shingled buildings":** Anne Morrow Lindbergh, *North to the Orient* (New York: Harcourt, Brace & Co., 1935), 124.

238 **By the 1960s, the sled dog population:** Coppinger, *World of Sled Dogs,* 76.

240 **"distance is over ten miles":** Coppinger and Coppinger, *Dogs: A New Understanding,* 157.

240 **"Siberians are kind of like":** Bob Thomas, International Siberian Husky Club, interview by the authors, June 2001.

Epilogue: End of the Trail

244 **"goaded on to the last"**: "Epic Struggle Brings Serum to End Plague," *San Francisco Chronicle*, February 3, 1925.

244 **"Science made the antitoxin"**: Editorial, *The New York Sun*, February 3, 1925.

244 **"that classic, heroic dog team"**: "Lauds Rescue Dogs in Senate Speech," *The New York Times*, February 7, 1925. Senator Dill's comments on the serum run from the Senate floor were widely reported in newspapers across the country.

245 **"in honor of Gunnar Kaasen's"**: Harry J. Harrcort to Bone, undated letter, National Archives, RG 90.

246 **"I was praying you'd be here"**: " 'Protect Me' Says Kassen, Nome's Hero," *Seattle Post-Intelligencer*, March 22, 1925.

247 **Balto sculpture unveiling**: "His Effigy Unveiled, Balto Is Unmoved," *The New York Times*, December 16, 1925.

247 **"He would rather make his hard mush"**: *Fairbanks Daily News-Miner*, February 9, 1925.

247 **"the shrinking modesty"**: *Seattle Post-Intelligencer*, March 22, 1925.

248 **"Nonsense," Kaasen snapped:** Tom Mahoney, "Arctic Dash Against Death," *Coronet Magazine* (October 1958).

248 **"in Alaska, our dogs mean"**: Ricker, *Alaskan Dog Driver*, 281.

248 **"It was almost more than"**: Ibid., 395.

249 **"I hope I shall never be"**: Ibid., 281.

250 **"They probably considered it"**: Thompson, *Seppala's Saga*, 2:36; Thompson wrote extensively about Seppala's tour through the states.

252 **"he had worked his hardest and his best"**: Ricker, *Alaskan Dog Driver*, 295.

252 **"It was a sad parting"**: Ibid.

252 **"Every once in a while a dog"**: "Dogs That Rank as Heroes Have a Hall of Fame," *The New York Times Magazine*, January 5, 1930.

252 **"in the depths of his keen gray eyes"**: Bruce Wilson, "The Champions of the Northland," n.d., Seppala Collection, Rasmuson.

253 **"While my trail has been rough"**: Thompson, *Seppala's Saga*, 2:60.

253 **He returned to Cleveland and began:** *Cleveland Plain Dealer* newspaper accounts, March 1927.

254 **"This hero business is big blah"**: Unidentified newspaper, Seppala Collection, Rasmuson.

254 **"I wouldn't take a million dollars"**: Churchill Fisher, "Lone Travelers in an Empty World," *Alaska Magazine* (November–December 1942).

255 **"I got more in gratitude"**: "Notes and Reviews," *Alaska Journal* (Spring 1979).

255 **"During the serum run I was"**: Matthew Donohue, "All in a Day's Work," *Alaska Magazine* (March 1980).

256 **"if the situation had not been so dire"**: T. A. Badger, "A Race to Save Lives," *Anchorage Daily News*, January 23, 1995.

256 **"I just wanted to help"**: "Edgar Nollner, 94, Dies; Musher in Alaska Relay," *The Washington Post*, January 20, 1999.

Appendix A

257 **"right and wrong"**: *Northland News* (September 1987).

258 **"I'm going to tell you this once"**: "Balto Film Triggers Memories of Musher," *The Herald* (Everett), January 9, 1995.

258 **"You had to be able to walk"**: *Edgar Kallands*, 53.

258 **"It made me feel good to know"**: Donohue, "All in a Day's Work," *Alaska Magazine* (March 1980).

258 **"A kind of normal operation"**: Ibid.

259 **"They pulled them three dead"**: Ibid.

259 **"smiling, hearty and proud"**: "Leonhard Seppala, Alaska Dog Team Champ," *Tacoma Sunday Ledger-News*, February 22, 1959.

260 **"In spite of his protestations"**: Lula Welch, "Northland Doctor's Wife."

261 **"the very commendable way"**: Surgeon General to Welch, April 11, 1925, Telegram, National Archives, RG 90.

261 **"Nome is on a slow retreat"**: Edward Curtis, Log Book, June Metcalf Collection, Rasmuson.

261 the town **"that would not die"**: Cole, *Nome: City of the Golden Beaches*, 161.

Selected Bibliography

Major Collections of Primary Sources

Alaska State Archives, Juneau
  Alaska Governor's Chronological Correspondence
  Alaska Territorial Government, Governor's Annual Reports
  Record Group 101, Territorial Governor's Office, General Correspondence, 1925

Alaska State Library, Juneau
  Governor Scott Bone Papers
  Mary Greene Papers

Carrie McLain Memorial Museum, Nome
  Diphtheria Folder, Daily Medical Reports
  Mark Summers Collection

Cleveland Museum Of Natural History
  Balto Exhibit Materials
  Mounted Balto, Cold Storage

International Siberian Husky Club, Elkorn, Wisconsin
  Breed's History
  Leonhard Seppala, personal papers

Kawerak, Inc. Native Corp., Nome
  Oral History Transcripts of Eskimos in Nome

Merck & Company, Archives, Whitehorse, New Jersey
  Company History and Antitoxin Products/Research and Development
  1925 Diphtheria Epidemic Files

National Archives, Washington, D.C.
    Department of the Interior, Governor's Correspondence, Record
      Group 348
    Records of the Judge Advocate General of the Navy, Navy Examining
      Boards 1890–1941, Record Group 125
    U.S. Public Health Service, General Correspondence, Record Group 90

Shelburne Museum, Shelburne, Vermont
    Togo Campaign for Return to Alaska Records

Siberian Husky Club Archives, Toronto, Canada

University of Alaska, Geophysical Institute, Fairbanks
    Weather Maps, Daily, January 1925–February 1925

University of Alaska, Rasmuson Library, Fairbanks
    Alaska Missions Collection
    Alaska Nurses Collection
    Iditarod Trail Oral History Project, Bureau of Land Management; 1980
      transcripts of interviews with surviving 1925 mushers (H83-16-
      15–H83-16-22)
    June Metcalf Collection
    William Mitchell Collection
    Leonhard Seppala Collection
    Daniel Sutherland Collection
    James Wickersham Collection

Yale University, New Haven, Connecticut
    Medical College Archives, Dr. Welch Personal File
    Peabody Museum Archives, Togo Taxidermy Records

Government Publications

Bureau of Land Management. *Iditarod National Historic Trail, Seward to Nome
    Route, A Comprehensive Management Plan.* Anchorage: U.S. Department
    of the Interior, 1986.
Bureau of Land Management. *Iditarod Trail Oral History Project* (tapes).
    Anchorage: U.S. Department of the Interior, 1980–81.
Central Intelligence Agency. *Polar Regions Atlas.* Washington, D.C.: CIA, 1978.
LaBelle, Joseph C., and James L. Wise. *Alaska Marine Ice Atlas.* Fairbanks:

Arctic Environmental Information and Data Center, University of Alaska, 1983.

United States Department of Commerce. *Coast and Geodetic Survey, United States Coast Pilot 9, Pacific and Arctic Coasts*, 7th edn. Washington, D.C.: Government Printing Office.

United States Department of Commerce, Weather Bureau. 1959. *Climates of the States: Alaska*. Washington, D.C.: Government Printing Office.

United States Department of Commerce, Weather Bureau. 1963. *Climatic Summary of Alaska: Supplement for 1922 Through 1952*. Washington, D.C.: Government Printing Office.

Principal Newspapers: 1925

Alaska Daily Empire
Anchorage Daily Alaskan
Anchorage Daily News
Anchorage Daily Times
Anchorage Weekly Alaskan
Chicago Daily Tribune
Cleveland Plain Dealer
Cleveland Press
Fairbanks Daily News-Miner
Los Angeles Times
The New York Evening Post
The New York Herald Tribune
The New York Sun
The New York Times
The New York World
Nome Daily Gold Digger
Nome Daily Nugget
Nome Nugget
San Francisco Chronicle
Seattle Daily Times
Seattle Post-Intelligencer
Seattle Sunday Times
Seattle Union Record
Tacoma News Tribune
Tacoma Times
Washington Herald
The Washington Post

Selected Bibliography

Books

Allan, Alexander. *Gold, Men and Dogs.* New York & London: G. P. Putnam's Sons, 1931.

Amundsen, Captain Roald. *The South Pole: An Account of the Norwegian Antartic Expedition in the Fram, 1910–1912.* New York: Cooper Square Press, 2001.

Berton, Pierre. *The Klondike Fever: The Life and Death of the Last Great Gold Rush.* New York: Carroll & Graf Publishers, 1985.

Bowers, Don. *Back of the Pack: An Iditarod Rookie Musher's Alaska Pilgrimage to Nome.* Anchorage: Publication Consultants, 1998.

Brooks, Alfred Hulse. *Blazing Alaska's Trails.* Fairbanks: University of Alaska Press, 1953.

Burch, Ernest S., Jr. *The Inupiaq Eskimo Nations of Northwest Alaska.* Fairbanks: University of Alaska Press, 1998.

Caldwell, Elsie Noble. *Alaska's Trail Dogs.* New York: Richard R. Smith, 1950.

Carrighar, Sally. *Moonlight at Midday.* New York: Alfred A. Knopf, 1967.

———. *Wild Voice of the North: The Chronicle of an Eskimo Dog.* New York: Doubleday & Company, 1959.

Cellura, Dominique. *Travelers of the Cold: Sled Dogs of the Far North.* Anchorage & Seattle: Alaska Northwest Books, 1989.

Chase, Allan. *Magic Shots.* New York: William Morrow & Co., 1982.

Colby, Merle. *A Guide to Alaska: Last American Frontier.* New York: The Macmillan Company, 1939.

Cole, Terrence. *Banking on Alaska: The Story of the National Bank of Alaska,* 2 vols. Anchorage: National Bank of Alaska, 2000.

———. *Crooked Past: The History of a Frontier Mining Camp: Fairbanks Alaska.* Alaska: University of Alaska Press, 1991.

———. *A History of the Nome Gold Rush: The Poor Man's Paradise.* PhD dissertation, University of Washington, 1983.

———. *Nome: City of the Golden Beaches.* Anchorage: Alaska Geographic Society, 1984.

Collins, Julie, and Miki Collins. *Trapline Twins.* Ancorage: Alaska Northwest Books, 1989.

Cook, Ann Mariah. *Running North: A Yukon Adventure.* Chapel Hill, NC: Algonquin Books of Chapel Hill, 1998.

Coppinger, Lorna. *The World of Sled Dogs: From Siberia to Sport Racing.* New York: Howell Book House, 1977.

Coppinger, Raymond, and Lorna Coppinger. *Dogs: A Startling New Under-*

standing *Of Canine Origin, Behavior and Evolution*. New York & London: Scribners, 2001.

Corbin, Wilford. *A World Apart: My Life Among the Eskimos of Alaska*. Alaska: Wizard Works, 2000.

Coren, Stanley. *The Intelligence of Dogs: A Guide to the Thoughts, Emotions, and Inner Lives of Our Canine Companions*. New York & London: Bantam Books, 1994.

Cushman, Dan. *The Great North Trail: America's Route of the Ages*, in American Trails series, ed. A. B. Guthrie, Jr. New York & London: McGraw-Hill Book Company, 1966.

Darling, Esther Birdsall. *Baldy of Nome*. Philadelphia: Penn Publishing Co., 1916.

———. *The Great Dog Races of Nome, Official Souvenir History* (1916). Knik, Alaska: Iditarod Trail Committee, 1969.

Davis, Mary Lee Cadwell. *We Are All Alaskans*. Boston: W. A. Wilde Co., 1931.

Deer, Mark. *Dog's Best Friend: Annals of the Dog-Human Relationship*. New York: Henry Holt & Company, 1997.

Demidoff, Lorna B. *The Complete Siberian Husky*. New York: Howell Book House, 1978.

Dufresne, Frank. *My Way Was North: An Alaskan Autobiography*. New York: Holt, Rinehart & Winston, 1966.

Edingtons, the. *Tundra: Romance and Adventure on Alaskan Trails*. New York: Grosset & Dunlap, 1930.

Fitzhugh, William W., and Aron Cromwell, eds. *Crossroads of Continents: Cultures of Siberia and Alaska*. Washington, D.C., & London: Smithsonian Institution Press, 1988.

Fitzhugh, William W., and Susan A. Kaplan. *Inua: Spirit World of the Bering Sea Eskimo*. Washington, D.C.: Smithsonian Institution Press, 1982.

Fortuine, Dr. Robert. *Chills & Fever: Health and Disease in the Early History of Alaska*. Fairbanks: University of Alaska Press, 1989.

Freedman, Lewis. *George Attla: The Legend of the Sled Dog Trail*. Harrisburg, PA: Stackpole Books, 1993.

Garst, Shannon. *Scotty Allan: King of the Dog-Team Drivers*. New York: Julian Messner, 1946.

Hammonds, Evelynn Maxine. *Childhood's Deadly Scourge: The Campaign to Control Diphtheria in New York City, 1880–1930*. Baltimore: Johns Hopkins University Press, 1999.

Harkey, Ira. *Pioneer Bush Pilot: The Story of Noel Wien*. Seattle: University of Washington Press, 1974.

Hunt, William R. *Arctic Passage: The Turbulent History of the Land and People of the Bering Sea 1697–1975*. New York: Charles Scribner's Sons, 1975.

———. *North of 53 Degrees: The Wild Days of the Alaskan-Yukon Mining Frontier 1870–1914*. New York: The Macmillan Company, 1974.

Huntford, Roland. *The Last Place on Earth*. New York: Atheneum, 1985.

Huntington, Sidney, as told to Jim Rearden. *Shadows on the Koyukuk*. Portland, OR: Alaska Northwest Books, 1993.

International Siberian Husky Club. *The Siberian Husky*, 3rd edn., ed. Pamela Thomas, Ann Stead, and Nancy Wolfe. Elkhorn, WI: International Siberian Husky Club, 1994.

Lindbergh, Anne Morrow. *North to the Orient*. New York: Harcourt, Brace & Company, 1935.

Lopez, Barry. *Arctic Dreams: Imagination and Desire in a Northern Landscape*. New York: Bantam Books, 1987.

Marshall, Max, ed. *The Story of the U.S. Army Signal Corps*. New York: Franklin Watts, 1965.

McLain, Carrie. *Gold Rush Nome*. Portland, OR: Graphic Arts Center, 1969.

Naske, Claus-M. *An Interpretative History of Alaskan Statehood*. Anchorage: Northwest Publishing Company, 1973.

Place, Marian T. *New York to Nome: The First International Cross-Country Flight*. New York: The Macmillan Company, 1972.

Poling, John. *A History of the Nome, Alaska Public Schools: 1899 to 1958; From the Gold Rush to Statehood*, master's thesis, University of Alaska, 1970.

Nelson, Edward William. *The Eskimos About Bering Strait*. Washington, D.C.: Smithsonian Institution Press, 1983.

Nelson, Richard K. *Hunters of the Northern Forest: Designs for Survival Among the Alaskan Kutchin*. Chicago & London: University of Chicago Press, 1973.

———. *Hunters of the Northern Ice*. Chicago & London: University of Chicago Press, 1969.

O'Brien, John. *Dog Sled for Byrd; 1600 Miles Across Antarctic Sea Ice*. Chicago: Thomas S. Rockwell Co., 1931.

O'Donoghue, Brian Patrick. *Honest Dogs: A Story of Triumph and Regret from the World's Toughest Sled Dog Race*. Portland, OR: Epicenter Press, 1999.

Oswalt, Wendell H. *Eskimos and Explorers*, 2nd edn. Lincoln & London: University of Nebraska Press, 1979.

Pease, Eleanor Fairchild. *Brave Tales of Real Dogs*. Chicago: Albert Whitman & Co., 1931.

Potter, Jean. *The Flying North: The Thrilling Story of the Bush Pilots in Alaska 1920–1945*. New York: Ballantine Books, 1945.

Ray, Dorothy Jean. *The Eskimos of Bering Strait, 1650–1898.* Seattle & London: University of Washington Press, 1975.

———. *Ethnohistory in the Arctic: The Bering Strait Eskimo,* ed. R. A. Pierce. Ontario: Limestone Press, 1983.

Reit, Seymour. *Race Against Death.* New York: Dodd, Mead & Co., 1976.

Renner, Louis, S.J. *Pioneer Missionary to the Bering Strait Eskimos: Bellarmine Lafortune, S.J.* Portland, OR: Binford & Mort, 1979.

Rennick, Penny, ed. *Dogs of the North.* Anchorage: Alaska Geographic Society, 1987.

Ricker, Elizabeth M., with Leonhard Seppala. *Seppala: Alaskan Dog Driver.* New York: Grosset & Dunlap, 1930.

———. *Togo's Fireside Reflections.* Lewiston, ME: Lewiston Journal Printshop, 1928.

Riddle, Maxwell, and Eva Seeley. *The Complete Alaskan Malamute.* New York: Howell Book House, 1976.

Riddles, Libby, and Tim Jones. *The Race Across Alaska.* Harrisburg, PA: Stackpole Books, 1988.

Roseberry, Cecil. *The Challenging Skies.* Garden City, NY: Doubleday & Company, 1966.

Schwartz, Marion. *A History of Dogs in the Early Americas.* New Haven: Yale University Press, 1997.

Scott, Alastair. *Tracks Across Alaska: A Dog Sled Journey.* New York: Atlantic Monthly Press, 1990.

Sherwonit, Bill. *Iditarod: The Great Race to Nome.* Anchorage: Northwest Books, 1991.

Smith, Herschel. *A History of Aircraft Piston Engines.* Manhattan, KS: Sunflower University Press, 1986.

Solka, Paul Jr., and Art Bremer. *Adventures in Alaska Journalism.* Fairbanks: Commercial Printing Co., 1980.

Stefansson, Vilhjalmur. *Arctic Manual.* Prepared under direction of the Chief of the Air Corps United States Army. New York: The Macmillan Company, 1957.

———. *The Friendly Arctic: The Story of Five Years in Polar Regions.* New York: The Macmillan Company, 1921.

———. *Hunters of the Great North.* New York: Harcourt, Brace & Company, 1922.

———. *My Life with the Eskimo.* New York: The Macmillan Company, 1922.

Stevens, Robert W. *Alaskan Aviation History.* Vol. 1: 1897–1928. Des Moines, WA: Polynyas Press, 1990.

Stuck, Hudson. *Ten Thousand Miles with a Dog Sled: A Narrative of Winter*

Travel in Interior Alaska. Lincoln & London: University of Nebraska Press, 1988.

Swenson, Olaf. *Northwest of the World: Forty Years Trading and Hunting in Northern Siberia.* New York: Dodd, Mead & Co., 1944.

Tabbert, Russ. *Dictionary of Alaskan English.* Juneau, AK: Denali Park, 1991.

Tanner, John Douglas, Jr. *Alaska Trails—Siberian Dogs.* Wheat Ridge, CO: Hoflin Publishing, 1986.

Thompson, Raymond. *Seppala's Saga of the Sled Dog,* 2 vols. Lynwood, WA, no publisher, 1977.

Ungermann, Kenneth A. *The Race to Nome: Alaska's Heroic Race to Save Lives.* Sunnyvale, CA: Press North America/Nulbay Associates, 1993.

Van der Linden, F. Robert. *Airlines and Air-Mail: The Post Office and the Birth of the Commercial Aviation Industry.* Kentucky: University Press of Kentucky, 2002.

Vaudrin, Bill. *Racing Alaskan Sled Dogs.* Anchorage: Alaska Northwest Publishing Co., 1976.

Vaughan, Norman D., with Cecil B. Murphy. *With Byrd at the Bottom of the World: The South Expedition of 1928–1930.* Harrisburg, PA: Stackpole Books, 1990.

Walden, Arthur T. *A Dog-Puncher on the Yukon.* Boston & New York: Houghton Mifflin Company, 1931.

Wickersham, James. *Old Yukon: Tales, Trails, Trials.* Washington, D.C.: Washington Law Book Company, 1938.

Willoughby, Barrett. *Alaskans All.* Boston & New York: Houghton Mifflin Company, 1933.

———. *Gentlemen Unafraid.* New York & London: G. P. Putnam's Sons, 1928.

Wirt, Loyal Lincoln. *Alaskan Adventures.* New York: Fleming H. Revell Co., 1937.

Wood, W. Barry. *Miasmas and Molecules.* New York & London: Columbia University Press, 1961.

Young, Edgerton. *My Dogs in the Northland.* London: S. W. Partridge & Co., 1902.

Yukon-Koyukuk School District of Alaska. *Bill McCarty, Sr.: A Biography.* Fairbanks: Spirit Mountain Press, 1982.

———. *Edgar Kallands: A Biography.* Fairbanks: Spirit Mountain Press, 1983.

Articles

Adams, Mildred. "Dogs That Rank As Heroes Have a Hall of Fame," *The New York Times Magazine,* January 3, 1930.

Akasofu, S.-I. "Aurora Borealis: The Amazing Northern Lights," *Alaska Geographic*, vol. 6, no. 2 (1979).

Beeson, Paul. "Rushing the Serum to the Rescue: A Long House Call," *Resident & Staff Physician* (April 1990).

Braafladt, O. A. "Men of Iron, Dogs of Speed," *Alaska Sportsman* (December 1937).

Caulfield, Ernest, M.D. "A True History of the Terrible Epidemic Vulgarly Called the Throat Distemper which occurred in His Majesty's New England Colonies Between the Years 1735–1740," *Yale Journal of Biology and Medicine* (1935).

Couch, Jim. "Fifty Years of Mushing," *Alaska Sportsman* (July 1958).

Donohue, Matthew. "All in a Day's Work: Mushers Recall Serum Run of 1925," *Alaska Magazine* (March 1980).

Dufresne, Frank. "The Greatest Dog Race the World Has Known," *Fairbanks Daily News-Miner*, February 26, 1927.

———. "Dog Mushing in Alaska," *Alaska Sportsman* (March 1936).

Kaiser, Henry. "Tracing a Tale of Mushing Heroism," *Fairbanks Daily News-Miner, Heartland*, February 3, 1985.

Lantis, Margaret. "Changes in the Alaskan Eskimo Relations of Man to Dog and Their Effects on Two Human Diseases," *Arctic Anthropology*, vol. XVII, no. 1 (1980).

Nelson, Jerry. "Perils of the Trail: Tales of Early Alaska and Yukon Mail Carriers," *Mushing Magazine* (January–February 1997).

Offen, Charlotte. "Angel of the Yukon," *True West* (March–April 1974).

Richardson, Jeffrey. "Serum Runner Remembers," *Senior Voice* (1986).

Seppala, Leonhard, with Raymond Thompson. "I Met My First Dog 60 Years Ago," *Alaska Sportsman* (May 1961).

———. "Nome Dog Races," *Alaska Sportsman* (July 1961).

———. "I Won the Nome Sweepstakes," *Alaska Sportsman* (November 1961).

———. "When Nome Needed Serum," *Alaska Sportsman* (May 1961).

———. "When Nome Needed Serum," *Alaska Sportsman* (January 1962).

Sharp, Henry S. "Man: Wolf: Woman: Dog," *Arctic Anthropology*, vol. XIII, no. 1 (1976).

Simpson, Sherry. "Heroes of the Mail Trail," *Alaska Magazine* (February 1996).

Smith, Lorne. "The Mechanical Dog Team: A Study of the Ski-Doo in the Canadian Arctic," *Arctic Anthropology*, vol. IX, no. 1 (1972).

Waller, Harold, as told to Charles Nadler. "The Alaska Tour of 1913," *Alaska Journal*, 16 (1986).

Welch, Lula, as told to Marion Rankin Kennedy. "Northland Doctor's Wife," parts 1–11, *Alaska Sportsman* (May 1965–May 1966).

West, Phoebe. "I Remember Nome," *Alaska Sportsman* (April 1962).

Wilcox, Marguerite Bone. "Memories of the Mansion," *Alaska Journal*, 16 (1986).

Willoughby, Barrett. "King of the Arctic Trails," *American Magazine* (August 1925).

———. "The Challenge of the Sweepstakes Trail," *American Magazine* (1926).

Select Interviews

Syun-Ichi Akasofu, Director, International Arctic Research Center, University of Alaska, Fairbanks, Alaska

Ed Blechner, Addison, Vermont

Susan Butcher, Fairbanks, Alaska

Charlie Campbell and Ruth Althoff, Tanana, Alaska

Elsie Chadwick, Siberian Husky Club, Toronto, Canada

Dermot Cole, Daily Columnist, *Fairbanks Daily News-Miner*

Professor Terrence Cole, Chair, History Department, University of Alaska, Fairbanks, Alaska

Ted Fathauer, Lead Forecaster, National Weather Service, Fairbanks, Alaska

Wendy Fitzgerald, Carp, Ontario

Dr. Robert Fortuine, Wasilla, Alaska

Bill Hanks and Sigrid Seppala-Hanks, Burlingame, California

Cussie Kauer, Nome, Alaska

Ruthmarie McDowell, Seattle, Washington

Steve Misencik, Cleveland Museum of Natural History, Cleveland, Ohio

Benoni Nelson, Knik Museum and Mushers Hall of Fame, Knik, Alaska

Dan O'Neill, Fairbanks, Alaska

Vesta Polsen, Hillsboro, Oregon

Donna Redding and Mike Zaidlic, Bureau of Land Management, Anchorage, Alaska

Penny Rennick, Alaska Geographic Society, Anchorage, Alaska

Sled Dog Museum and Iditarod Headquarters, Wasilla, Alaska

Jerry A. Steiger, Meteorologist, National Weather Service, Nome, Alaska

Jack Strege, Everett, Arizona

Dr. Bill Stringer, Professor Emeritus, Geophysical Institute, University of Alaska, Fairbanks, Alaska

Pam and Bob Thomas, International Siberian Husky Club, Elkhorn, Wisconsin

Dirk Tordoff, Film Archivist, University of Alaska, Fairbanks, Alaska
Kenneth A. Ungermann, St. Augustine, Florida
Jona Van Zyle, Eagle River, Alaska
Ann Walsh of Fairbanks, Alaska; Jim and Betty Walsh of Seattle, Washing-
    ton; Joe Walsh of Fairbanks, Alaska
Janice Weiland, Arlington, Virginia
Jean Summers-Wolf, San Francisco
Dale and Nancy Wolff, Dayton, Ohio

Web Sites

www.akc.org (The American Kennel Club)
www.anchorage.ak.blm.gov/inht3.html (Bureau of Land Management's
    Iditarod National Historic Trail)
www.iditarod.com (Iditarod Trail Committee)
www.ckcusa.com/seppala/isssc.htm (International Seppala Siberian Sled
    Dog Club)
www.ckcusa.com/seppala/isssc.htm (Leonhard Seppala's geneology)
www.gi.alaska.edu (Geophysical Institute, University of Alaska, Fairbanks)
http://home.no.net/tunheim/seppala/seppalae.htm (Leonhard Seppala's
    history in Norway)
www.iarc.uaf.edu (International Arctic Research Center)
www.ishclub.org/history.html (International Siberian Husky Club)
www.mnh.si.edu/arctic/features/croads/eskimo.html (Arctic Studies Center
    of the Smithsonian National Museum of Natural History)
www.nomekennelclub.com (Nome Kennel Club)
www.nomenugget.com (*Nome Nugget*, Alaska's oldest newspaper)
www.theserumrun.com (Colonel Vaughan's Annual Commemorative Run)
www.troms-slekt.com/historical/kaasen/gkmain.htm (Gunnar Kaasen's
    genealogy)